WHAT EVERY WOMAN SHOULD KNOW

STAYING HEALTHY AFTER 40

WHAT EVERY WOMAN SHOULD KNOW

STAYING HEALTHY AFTER 40

LILA NACHTIGALL, M.D.,
ROBERT D. NACHTIGALL, M.D.
AND JOAN RATTNER HEILMAN

WARNER BOOKS

A Time Warner Company

Warner Books, Inc., 1271 Avenue of the Americas, New York, NY 10020

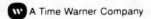 A Time Warner Company

Printed in the United States of America
First Printing: July 1995
10 9 8 7 6 5 4 3 2 1

Library of Congress Cataloging-in-Publication Data

Nachtigall, Lila.
    What every woman should know: staying healthy after 40 / Lila
Nachtigall, Robert Nachtigall, and Joan Rattner Heilman.
        p.   cm.
    Includes index.
    ISBN 0-446-51731-3
    1. Middle aged women—Health and hygiene.   I. Nachtigall, Robert.
II. Heilman, Joan Rattner. III. Title.
RA778.N24 1995
613'.04244—dc20   94-32695
                                                                          CIP

Book design by Giorgetta Bell McRee

Dedicated to:

The four generations of wonderful women in our families: ranging from Grammy approaching 90 to Julia Celene approaching 1 year.

Acknowledgments

Our special thanks to three physicians who provided invaluable assistance in the research for this book:

Wendy Keller Epstein, M.D., Assistant Clinical Professor of Dermatology, New York University School of Medicine;

Richard H. Nachtigall, M.D., Professor of Clinical Medicine, New York University School of Medicine; and

Bertrand Agus, M.D., Associate Professor of Clinical Medicine, New York University School of Medicine.

Contents

Chapter 1

STAY HEALTHIER, FEEL YOUNGER, LIVE LONGER

IF YOU WANT TO LIVE a healthier, longer life, this book is for you. Written to answer all of the questions we have heard over and over again in our many years of practice as specialists in women's health, it is designed as an accessible, easy-to-read guide to the special concerns of women over 40.

It will give you the latest scientific information on keeping your skin young and vibrant, your figure within bounds, your sex life on track, and your uterus and ovaries intact. It will help you protect yourself against heart disease and bone fractures. It will provide the most recent data on reducing the risk of breast cancer, getting through menopause with ease, making a decision about hormone replacement therapy, avoiding vaginitis and urinary-tract infections, dealing with fibroids, coping with uncooperative bladders, choosing a contraceptive, even having a baby in your forties.

In sum, this book is designed to help you keep your body in optimum working order for the rest of your life. It will allow you to have some control over your future.

None of us is going to live forever—nor do we want to—but we all want to spend our lives in the best possible shape.

1

We want to grow older in good health and good style, unhampered by bodies that can't keep up with us. Unlike a century ago, when few women survived beyond 50, we are living longer than ever before. Most of us at 40- or 50-something have over half of our lives yet to go; and there's no reason not to get through it all with zest, flair, and enthusiasm.

As the biggest and best-educated midlife generation to come along so far—the women who flocked to childbirth classes and clamored to take part in their own health decisions—most of today's over-40 women are intensely interested in the workings of their bodies and eager to take responsibility for keeping them in good operating condition. What's more, we are starting to understand that there's more to staying healthy than good genes and good luck. It also requires a few sensible changes in lifestyle and some practical measures that can make anyone of any age, despite years of careless living, a lot healthier.

Today we have some control over how we age. There's much we can do to postpone, minimize, or even prevent what used to be considered the inevitable consequences of time, but are actually due to unhealthy habits, disease, and environmental wear-and-tear. Right now, you are faced with the perfect opportunity to make an assessment of your health and your habits. The choices you make today can have a powerful effect on the quality of your life tomorrow.

IT'S *YOUR* BODY

Now is the time when you can have the greatest positive effect on your future health. As a woman who's heading into the middle years or is already in them, you are looking at your very last chance to stave off the most dire effects of aging, preserve your youthful body, prevent or delay many diseases, and offer yourself the chance of living a longer, healthier life. When you were 20 or 30, you could get away with almost any unhealthy behavior, but now you are losing your margin for error. Poor health habits can be much more damaging and much less reversible than they were when you were younger, making prevention increasingly important.

And that's what this book is all about: how to take positive steps now so you won't have to worry later. A guide to the most common health problems faced by women over 40, its aim is to give you the latest information, all of the available facts, the newest thinking about what is happening to your body, and the valid medical options for keeping yourself fit and healthy over the long term.

After all, it's *your* body. You are the one who knows it best, the one with the most to gain by taking care of it. Take charge! Fight back! Defend your body against the ravages of time and all its avoidable illnesses and mishaps. Do what you can now to keep your body working well later. Don't wait for things to go wrong before you step in. Prevent them from happening before they do. In other words, start practicing preventive maintenance now.

ALTERING ATTITUDES

The thinking about health and medicine has changed radically in just the last few years. As recently as a decade ago, for example, most of us thought of exercise merely as the route to a better-looking body. Today we look beyond the superficial results to its more important, long-term health benefits. For years we considered food almost completely in terms of calories, but now we know that the right nutrients can prevent disease and prolong our lives. Medicine has always been the way to make us better when we got sick, but today we are beginning to understand that it can also help prevent illness and disabilities before they ever happen.

When a good night's sleep begins to sound more inviting than a night on the town, you have entered a new phase of your physiological life. Although questions of contraception, fertility, and PMS may still linger in your mind, new and threatening subjects such as menopause, heart disease, brittle bones, and liver spots are becoming more crucial issues. If you are reading this book, you have already taken the first step in preparing for this next phase. You have started educating yourself, taking charge of your own body, and anticipating the future. The more knowledge you can acquire and the more understanding you can gain about the many issues of growing older, the more control you will have over the second half of your life.

The older we get, the more obvious it becomes that not all people age at the same rate. Some women are obviously much younger than others at the same chronological age. Some at 60 or 70 or even beyond 90 remain energetic, attractive, fit, vibrant, and productive, while others march alongside the biological clock or even ahead of it. Some of the variations come from genetic differences but much emanates from life-long lifestyles. The truth is that the number of years you have lived is not nearly as important as how well you have maintained your body over time.

Use this book as a maintenance manual for your body, letting you know what to expect, what's normal and what's not, and what you can do about both. Use it to find the answers to all of your questions about how to live a longer, healthier life.

Chapter 2

PERIMENOPAUSE: TIME OF TRANSITION

IT'S AROUND THEIR FORTIETH BIRTHDAY that most women today start to realize they are no longer among the young and resilient and begin to focus on the effects that age will have on their lives. It is also the time when some very subtle changes start taking place in their bodies. These changes are called *perimenopause*.

A strange and confusing period of time for many women, perimenopause begins when your ovaries' production of estrogen and progesterone, the two major female hormones, starts to diminish significantly. It ends at menopause, your last menstrual period. A normal and natural process, perimenopause signals a new phase of physiological life, and so it offers the perfect time to prepare for menopause and its potential effects on your emotions, your bones, your heart, your bladder, and even your sex life.

Most women start noticing the signs of perimenopause a year or two before they stop menstruating, although for some, menopause can be many years—perhaps as many as eight or ten—in their future. The average age for menopause in the United States is 52, with a normal range of 45 to 55. But don't count on that. Approximately eight out of a hundred women in this country have a natural menopause before the age of 40, and others have an early and abrupt "surgical" menopause because of outside intervention such as surgery, radiation, or chemotherapy. At the other end of the spectrum, five out of every hundred women menstruate until they're almost 60.

All women can benefit enormously from knowing what's going on in their bodies and how to best deal with those changes.

WHAT YOU CAN DO *NOW*

You can prepare now for the future by eating properly, exercising, getting routine checkups, and quitting bad habits such as smoking.

If you haven't been having regular physical and gynecological examinations, it is essential to begin right now. Make an appointment for a complete checkup, which includes a mammogram, a breast exam, a Pap smear, a cardiogram, a stool test, bone-density measurements if you are a prime candidate for osteoporosis, estrogen and/or follicle-stimulating hormone (FSH) measurements, cholesterol measurements, and other urine and blood tests that provide baselines against which future changes can be compared. In most cases it is best to see a gynecologist for this checkup, or at least part of it, because this is the physician who has had special training in women's health issues.

PERIMENOPAUSE EXPLAINED

Estrogen, the major female hormone, is responsible for the physical changes during puberty that turn a young girl's body into a woman's. Estrogen combines with *progesterone*, the second most important female hormone, to prepare the body for conception and pregnancy. After puberty, tiny fluid-filled sacs called *follicles* develop in the ovaries every month, releasing an egg into the fallopian tube on its way to the uterus, in a process called *ovulation*.

Meanwhile, the lining of the uterus, under the influence of estrogen and progesterone, builds up into a thickened tissue ready to support a fertilized egg and a developing fetus. When the egg is not fertilized and conception does not occur, progesterone triggers the shedding of that thick lining—the *endometrium*—during the next menstrual period.

These cyclical events begin to change as your body approaches menopause. It's rather like puberty in reverse. The ovaries have a finite supply of follicles that ripen into eggs. Two or three years before menopause, you have depleted most of them and stop ovulating. With just a few viable follicles left, you produce eggs irregularly or only occasionally, and, as a result, your production of progesterone diminishes and your periods become erratic and irregular. Some months you bleed profusely, others hardly at all. Sometimes you skip a month or two, or your periods arrive very early or very late. Sometimes they vanish for several months, then return for several more. Without a regular supply of progesterone, the endometrium is shed at random.

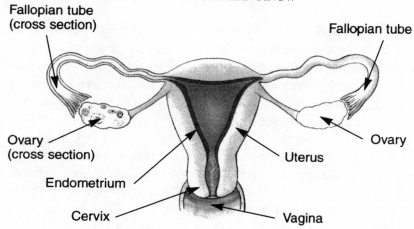

Fallopian tube
(cross section)

Fallopian tube

Ovary
(cross section)

Ovary

Uterus

Endometrium

Cervix

Vagina

"I never know what to expect. One month I have a very heavy period, the next practically nothing. Some months I have no period at all or it's very late or it lasts almost two weeks. Is this normal?"

It certainly is. Almost every possible variation is normal. Although some women simply stop menstruating one day and that is that, most are never sure what is going to happen next. This unsettling phase may last only a few months or it may go on for several years. But the average duration is a year or two.

"I worry that something's wrong when I have unexpected bleeding, even though I'm the right age for menopause. How do I handle this?"

See your gynecologist. Any irregular or different bleeding should always be checked out. Although the cause may well be perimenopause, there's a chance that it isn't. Your gynecologist will probably suggest an endometrial biopsy, a dilatation and curettage (D & C), or perhaps ultrasound to rule out the remote possibility of cancer, and then will continue to monitor your periods with periodic exams after that. In the meantime be sure to report any new developments. You are having erratic periods because you are not ovulating at all or only occasionally and therefore you no longer produce enough progesterone to stimulate the regular monthly shedding of the uterine lining. Meanwhile, however, you still manufacture estrogen, which thickens the lining as always in anticipation of a possible pregnancy.

"Is there anything to do about these irregular periods except endure them?"

Because unexpected bleeding can be unnerving, you may elect to get your periods back on a comfortably predictable schedule by supplying the missing progesterone in a cyclical pattern. You can do this by taking progesterone alone, usually given as Provera in doses of 5 to 10 milligrams daily for ten to twelve days every four (or eight) weeks, to keep the bleeding under control and give you regular periods again until menopause. These periods begin within a few days after you've taken your last progesterone pill of the cycle.

The cyclical progesterone will also ensure that the endometrium is completely shed every month. Very often, because of the diminished production of progesterone during perimenopause, the uterine lining is not sloughed off as thoroughly as it should be.

Another benefit is that now you can avoid frequent biopsies. Because irregular bleeding must always be monitored to be sure nothing more worrisome than perimenopause is going on, your doctor will undoubtedly suggest periodic biopsies of the endometrium (uterine lining) so the tissues can be examined for the presence of abnormal cells. However, when the hormone treatment verifies that your erratic bleeding was caused by a progesterone deficiency, you won't need so many biopsies because now you will be bleeding according to plan.

An alternative way to regulate your periods is to take low-dose combination oral contraceptives. Not only will the pill restore your periods to a regular monthly pattern but it will simultaneously relieve symptoms such as hot flashes and prevent pregnancy. (See next question.) The newest oral contraceptives contain much lower doses of hormones than their predecessors, and unlike the older varieties, do not encourage heart attacks or strokes in healthy women. They have recently been approved by the FDA for women up to the age of 50.

"I know you skip periods when you're going into menopause but how do I know I'm not pregnant? I have fairly regular periods for a few months, then I skip a month or two or have them six or seven weeks apart. I am 43 with two grown children, and I definitely do not want to have another baby."

There's always the remote chance that a skipped period means you are pregnant. It happens to many 43-year-old women, delighting only a few of them. If you have any reason to suspect that this could be true, ask your doctor to give you a pregnancy test. Even though your chances for pregnancy drop dramatically during your forties, you never know when you are going to produce one last egg, and all it takes is one energetic sperm to change your life. To eliminate even the most remote chance that you will get pregnant, continue to use contraception now and for at least six months after menopause.

"What's the best kind of birth control for women who are in the perimenopause stage?"

You are safe in choosing any of several methods of contraception (see Chapter 9), but the low-dose combination birth-control pills, which contain only small amounts of estrogen and progesterone, may be your best answer *if* you are not a smoker. This method, as we have explained, will not only prevent pregnancy but regulate your periods and suppress early menopausal symptoms at the same time. You will no longer have to wonder whether a skipped period means you're pregnant because you won't be skipping any.

Building Your Bones for the Future

Now is your last chance to build your bones before menopause, when you start losing a large percentage of bone mass. Here's how to do it:

- Consume enough calcium (at least 1,000 milligrams per day before menopause, 1,500 after) from food and/ or supplements.
- Get enough weight-bearing exercise, which means at least a half hour of moderate activity three times a week.

If you are not planning to take hormone replacement therapy (HRT) after menopause, have bone-density measurements taken now to provide a baseline against which future measurements can be compared (see Chapter 4). Bone loss begins in the spine, sometimes even before menopause, so don't settle for measurements of the cortical bone in your wrists or hips only. Then, have another set of measurements made a year after menopause. This will give you an estimate of your percentage of bone loss per year. Some women lose only 1 or 2 percent a year and probably don't have to be concerned about osteoporosis, while others lose 8 or 10 percent annually after menopause. If you are in the latter group, you can't afford to do that for very long. See Chapter 4 for more about your bones.

"I am obviously in perimenopause because my periods are very strange, but I don't have any menopausal symptoms yet. When do they usually start?"

Most women don't have the typical menopausal symptoms such as hot flashes and palpitations during perimenopause, but get them after their estrogen has dropped so low that they no longer have periods at all. In 15 to 20 percent of women, however, the symptoms begin earlier.

"I am still having regular periods, but I have bad hot flashes. What can I do about them?"

Try taking daily doses of vitamin E, which may keep your perimenopausal hot flashes under control. Start with 400 units twice a day, and if you have no results after about a week, double the dose for a daily total of 1,600 units. You can't possibly get that much of this vitamin in your daily diet, so you'll have to take supplements.

And you may wish to take vitamins B and C supplements, too, because, although there is no scientific proof of their effectiveness, some women swear they work. Start with one B-50 tablet and 500 milligrams of vitamin C a day.

The next step that we usually recommend to healthy non-smoking women is to go on the pill—the new low-dose kind. It may be just what you need. The thinking has changed about the safety of taking estrogen before menopause, and besides, the pill is not what it used to be. In the past it was believed dangerous to take supplemental estrogen in any form before menopause because it could cause hyperplasia, an excessive buildup of the endometrium that can be a precancerous condition.

But recent studies have shown that it is safe to prescribe estrogen in the form of low-dose combination birth-control pills for women in perimenopause, and the FDA has approved it for women up to the age of 50. The pill can make this difficult phase much more tolerable by alleviating early menopausal symptoms. At the same time, it keeps your periods regular *and* solves the pregnancy problem. The pill does have potential side effects, however, such as breast tenderness, weight gain, water retention, and depression. If you find these are only minimally bothersome, you have found an easy way out of a lot of difficulties.

A newly approved contraceptive, Depo-Provera, is another way to alleviate hot flashes and other uncomfortable perimenopausal symptoms in women who can't take estrogen, or for religious reasons don't want to take the pill, although it can make your periods even more irregular and may have PMS-like side effects. All progesterone with no estrogen, it is taken by injection every three months, which means its side effects may last at least three months, too.

"I remember that some women couldn't take the pill in the old days because it caused blood clots. So, what's different now?"

The amount of estrogen in the pill is so low now (although higher than the dosage in hormone replacement therapy) that it is considered safe as long as you don't have a history of serious clotting problems or are a smoker. Recent data suggest that the pill reduces the risk of both uterine and ovarian cancer. In addition, ovarian cysts, benign fibrocystic breast disease, and dysmenorrhea (painful menstrual periods) are less common among pill users.

"If it's safe to take the pill before menopause, why can't I take estrogen-replacement therapy instead?"

You can, but you may be better served by birth-control pills. In perimenopause, hormone replacement therapy is usually reserved for women who suffer from severe symptoms, have tried other means of dealing with them, and can't tolerate birth-control pills. That's because, during this transitional phase, you may periodically produce high levels of your own estrogen, and you don't want to add more unless necessary. Besides, the pill combines estrogen and progesterone in one handy tablet and prevents pregnancy.

"If I take the low-dose birth-control pills and have regular periods again, how will I know when I have menopause?"

You won't, unless you stop taking the pills and have your follicle-stimulating hormone (FSH) level measured. This is a simple blood test that measures the amount of the hormone, a substance that increases as your estrogen level falls. But it really doesn't matter because the hormones in the pill will have protected you from osteoporosis and probably cardiovascular disease, just as hormone replacement therapy would have done. At age 50, you can stop and either wait for telltale hot flashes or have your FSH measured, and then switch to hormone replacement therapy if you want to.

Danger! No Smoking!

If you are a smoker, do not use birth-control pills, low-dose or otherwise. The pill exaggerates smokers' already considerable risk of heart attack and stroke.

"I have a friend who says she has no trouble with hot flashes because she drinks a special Chinese herbal tea. What's your opinion of that?"

Some women find that plant materials like ginseng, dong quai, spirulina, sage, wild yam, licorice, sassafras, and linseed help relieve hot flashes. The truth is that these herbal remedies sometimes work for symptoms that aren't too severe. Some of them, in fact, are potent sources of plant estrogen, and therefore are actually a kind of estrogen-replacement therapy. Not chemically the same as the human hormone but structurally similar, these vegetable estrogens, known as phytoestrogens—especially ginseng and dong quai—can produce a demonstrable biological response.

However, although these plant materials are natural, which for many women makes them preferable to prescribed drugs, there is no way to control the amount of estrogen they provide. So unless they are taken in combination with progesterone to protect the uterine lining, it is possible for them to cause hyperplasia, an excessive buildup of the tissue that may eventually lead to cancer. Our advice is to treat them just as cautiously as you would prescription medicines.

An alternative to using phytoestrogens as medicine is to increase your consumption of fruits and vegetables, many of which, especially soybean products, contain natural estrogen.

"In the last few months, I've developed PMS for the first time in my life. What's happening?"

PMS remains a mystery, for which no one yet has a good answer. Sometimes women who have suffered from PMS their entire adult lives find that it disappears at perimenopause. But for others, it gets much worse during this transitional time. And for still others—women who never ever had PMS before—this is the time it first makes its appearance.

We don't know for sure what causes PMS, but it probably is related to ovarian hormones and perhaps to the ratio of estrogen to progesterone. Studies have shown that when estrogen levels fall below a certain point, symptoms of anxiety and depression are common. What may be happening is that the ovaries now produce less estrogen than they once did, while at the same time, you continue to ovulate and manufacture normal amounts of progesterone. Progesterone—well known for making some women feel nervous, irritable, and anxious—may overpower the decreased estrogen and result in PMS symptoms.

"What can I do to relieve the PMS?"

Try increasing your fluid intake, cutting down on salt, and taking vitamin B_6 (no more than 500 milligrams per day), a natural diuretic. Or for cyclical weight gain, bloating, or breast tenderness, try taking Aldactone, a mild diuretic. Also step up your calcium consumption. Government researchers have found that women who consume at least 1,300 mg of calcium a day have significantly fewer problems with mood swings as well as with "aches and pains."

Other potentially helpful measures include relaxation techniques, tranquilizers, and a daily diet low in fat and sugar and high in fiber and complex carbohydrates.

Another solution is to take estrogen supplements for two weeks before your menstrual periods. Most women feel better when their estrogen level is above a certain level, usually about 50 picograms per milliliter. Other medications, usually with side effects of their own, can also be prescribed by your gynecologist.

And last, perhaps birth-control pills are your answer. Substituting a fixed daily dose of estrogen and synthetic progesterone for the ovaries' monthly fluctuations, they offer the possibility of an easy, low-cost way of eliminating PMS.

"My periods are still very regular, and as I'm only 40, I doubt I'm about to have menopause. However, I do find that my vagina is getting dryer and sex has become uncomfortable. I use a lubricant before intercourse. Any other suggestions?"

Vaginal dryness usually doesn't become a problem until a few years after a woman stops making estrogen, but everybody's different.

The first thing to try is one of the over-the-counter vaginal moisturizing gels such as Replens or Gyne-Moistrin, which moisturize the cells of the vaginal lining, making it less dry and irritable. Used regularly about three times a week, they usually do a good job.

If the moisturizers don't restore the vaginal tissues well enough to make intercourse comfortable, the next step is a low-dose vaginal estrogen cream that's applied a few times a week. Although this is actually a form of estrogen replacement and requires a prescription, very little of the hormone is absorbed into the bloodstream once the tissues of the vaginal lining have been restored to good working order.

During intercourse, use an over-the-counter vaginal lubricant such as K-Y Jelly as well. Never use a lubricant (especially petroleum jelly) that is not designed specifically for this purpose, because it can make matters a lot worse by irritating the tissues, caking, or blocking your own secretions. And never use a vaginal moisturizing gel as a lubricant. It doesn't work as well as a lubricant, which is designed to make things easier during intercourse; but even more important, a vaginal moisturizer has a low pH, which means it is acidic, helpful in fighting off unwanted bacteria. Applied to your vagina just before intercourse, it can be very irritating to your partner's delicate tissues. For more about sex, see Chapter 7.

"Is there any way to tell how close you are to menopause?"

Yes, by testing the follicle-stimulating hormone (FSH) level of your blood on the second or third day after your menstrual period begins. The higher the level, the closer you are to menopause. There is a hormonal relationship between the pituitary gland, which produces FSH, and the ovaries, which make estrogen. As the ovaries reduce their output of estrogen, the pituitary gland senses it and turns out more and more FSH in an effort to get the ovaries going again. The less estrogen, the more FSH.

So if you are truly in perimenopause and menopause is just over the horizon, not only will your estrogen level be lower but your FSH will be higher. In normal premenopausal women, the FSH level in your blood is usually about 10 micro international units per milliliter (mIU/ml). When it rises to 20 or 25 mIU/ml, you are definitely perimenopausal. At 40 mIU/ml, you no longer have to wonder. Your periods will usually stop, and it will be clear that you have reached menopause.

FSH levels tend to rise gradually and seldom retreat, so it

is useful to compare them over time if you want to make a prediction. If, for example, you have a level of 16 mIU/ml today and 30 mIU/ml next year, you probably won't have long to wait for menopause.

FSH levels can also be useful in predicting the chances of achieving pregnancy among women over 40 who want to have a baby (see Chapter 10). An FSH level of 20 mIU/ml or more means that pregnancy is most unlikely. Over 25 mIU/ml, the possibilities are close to zero. Because the FSH level varies with your menstrual cycle, you will be tested on one of the first three days of your period, when estrogen is at its lowest point.

"I have very large fibroids that cause heavy bleeding, and I've been told to do nothing about them now because they will shrink after menopause. Do you agree with that?"

It all depends on their size, how fast they are growing, how much hemorrhaging or pressure they cause, and how close you are to menopause. Fibroids—uterine muscle tumors that are benign 99 percent of the time—are most common among women in their early forties, although sometimes they occur before that. If you are not close to menopause and you are still producing a lot of estrogen, they will continue to grow. Another reason to measure your FSH.

If your FSH is low, indicating you are not going to have menopause very soon, and your fibroids are causing major problems, you may have to consider having them removed surgically by myomectomy or hysterectomy. If your FSH is high, meaning that menopause is just down the road, and you are not losing tremendous amounts of blood, you can wait to see if the symptoms subside as your estrogen level drops.

By the way, you may want to think about using low-dose combination oral contraceptives. Unlike the higher-dose pills of the past, they often encourage fibroids to shrink, decreasing the heavy bleeding.

Finally, Menopause

When you have had no menstrual periods, erratic or otherwise, for at least six consecutive months, you can safely conclude that you've reached menopause. Your doctor can confirm this by measuring your FSH level. Over 40 mIU/ml (it can go all the way up to 1,000), and the answers are in.

Chapter 3

MENOPAUSE: A PHYSIOLOGICAL CHANGE

MENOPAUSE, ONLY RECENTLY OUT OF THE CLOSET, has become one of the leading women's health issues of the nineties. With life expectancy steadily lengthening, millions of baby boomers maturing, and a well-educated generation of women seeking to understand their bodies, women want to know everything about this physiological happening and how it can affect their health and their lives. Although the average age for menopause in the United States is 52, many women experience it even before they are 40, so it is never too soon to investigate this normal female biological process so you can deal with it intelligently.

Nor is it ever too late after menopause to take action in behalf of your own well-being. A newborn girl today can expect to live to almost 80, while a woman who has reached the age of 40 or 50 in good health may live well beyond 90. It certainly makes sense to live those extra years feeling good.

WHAT YOU CAN DO *NOW*

Find out what's going on in your body around the time of menopause and what, if anything, you should do about it. There are important decisions to be made, most especially whether to take hormone replacement therapy. There are arguments both pro and con, and the results of new research appear in the press almost daily. You will surely need to sort fact from theory, so we will do our best to help you do that right here.

To start, talk to your female relatives about your family's menopausal history because you will most likely follow familial patterns. Find a doctor, preferably a gynecologist, who keeps current with developments in menopause management and encourages you to take part in making decisions about your own body.

Meanwhile:

- Stop smoking.
- Limit your alcohol intake.
- Consume adequate calcium.
- Get enough vitamin D from sun or milk.
- Eat well-balanced low-fat meals.
- Get plenty of exercise.
- Quit going on drastic diets.

WHEN WILL IT HAPPEN?

The average age for menopause in the United States is 52, with most women having their last menstrual periods between the ages of 45 and 55. About five out of every hundred women continue to menstruate regularly after 53, some even as late as 60 or more. And eight out of every hundred women have a spontaneous menopause before 40.

Your age at menopause is determined almost exclusively by your genes and has no relationship to the age at which you had your first period. So without outside intervention, you can count on having menopause at about the same time your mother and maternal grandmother did.

Of course, you will have instant menopause at any age if your ovaries are surgically removed or severely damaged by radiation or chemotherapy. And you may have it earlier than expected, maybe even five years earlier, if you are a heavy smoker.

YOUR CHANGING BODY

Menopause is the time when menstruation ends forever. It is your very last menstrual period, the transition from the reproductive to the nonreproductive stage of your life. Your estrogen production began tapering off in your thirties, and your lifetime supply of egg follicles has gradually been depleted, so that in your forties or fifties you no longer have eggs to release or estrogen to stimulate ovulation and monthly periods.

Although you continue to make small amounts of estrogen in your ovaries and fat tissue even after menopause, you no longer have enough of it to be fertile or have menstrual periods. As a result, many things happen in your body, some of them typical of *every* woman at menopause over the long term. Other effects are simply responses to your new low levels of female hormones, and are temporary and infinitely variable. These are the infamous menopausal symptoms that can last for years and may make your life miserable, but that will eventually fade away.

THE VARIABLES:
MENOPAUSAL SYMPTOMS

Everybody's different, and at menopause, that statement couldn't be more true. Some women hardly notice they've had menopause except that they stop having menstrual periods. Others have such uncomfortable symptoms that they can hardly function. And between the extremes are the majority of women whose symptoms range from insignificant to miserable. Symptoms may include not only the well-known hot flashes and night sweats but many other equally strange happenings that can be disturbing or even frightening if you aren't prepared for them.

The classic menopausal symptoms:

- Hot flashes and night sweats
- Palpitations
- Insomnia
- Tingling or "pins and needles"
- Intermittent numbness, especially in your fingers
- Dizziness
- Joint and muscle pains
- Mood changes
- Irritability, depression, fatigue, tension, anxiety
- Formication or "crawling" skin
- Shortness of breath
- Headaches
- Dry eyes
- Dry mouth, "burning" mouth
- Altered taste perception
- Forgetfulness

Some women never have any of these symptoms. Probably no woman ever has all of them. But at least 75 percent have hot flashes or other disturbances to one degree or another. If you have them, remember that you are absolutely normal and that these odd events are not figments of your imagination. Menopause symptoms simply are the tangible signs of a measurable hormonal event that happens to every woman who lives long enough to have menopause. They are absolutely harmless, and whether or not you treat them, they will almost always fade away when your body adjusts to its new hormone levels.

FAST FACTS ABOUT HOT FLASHES

Hot flashes are sudden feelings of heat that sweep over your entire body but especially your upper body, face, and neck. Your skin temperature may be measurably elevated and your pulse rate slightly accelerated. Your skin becomes flushed and may break out in red blotches. In most cases you sweat profusely at the same time.

When your estrogen level falls, the pituitary gland produces vast amounts of follicle-stimulating hormone (FSH) in an effort to persuade the ovaries to get back to work making estrogen again. The high levels of this pituitary hormone, together with increased activity of a part of the brain called the hypothalamus, cause your normal temperature-regulating mechanisms to over-react. It is now known that the hypothalamus has estrogen receptors that, left unsatisfied, respond by releasing substances much like epinephrine and result in these *vasomotor* events that affect the peripheral blood vessels.

• Flashes and sweating are usually worse at night, waking some women up five or six times a night so drenched that they may have to change their night-clothes or even their sheets.

- Sometimes there's a warning feeling or "aura" that signals an oncoming hot flash.
- The intense heat wave is usually followed by chills and a feeling of constriction of the skin that may last for several hours.
- Hot flashes can last anywhere from a few brief moments to more than an hour. Some are hardly noticeable while others are acutely uncomfortable. Some women have only a few mild episodes a day, while others experience forty or fifty severe flashes in the same period of time.
- For about half of all women, the symptoms taper off and vanish within a year. For about a third, they persist for up to two and a half years. And for the remaining 20 percent, they last for five, ten, or twenty years—or, for an unlucky few, for the rest of their lives.
- Most women experience no hot flashes until their estrogen level is very low, their FSH level is very high, and menopause is a documented event, but others may have them long before that.

"What causes menopausal symptoms like palpitations and tingling fingers?"

All of the temporary symptoms result from vasomotor instability and are considered the equivalent of hot flashes.

"Sometimes I get this weird crawling sensation on my skin. I am hoping it is a menopausal symptom that will go away eventually."

It is formication, a typical though rather rare menopausal symptom and probably the strangest one of all. Eventually it will disappear on its own. If you don't want to wait that long, you'll find that estrogen replacement can put a quick end to it.

"I have been having periods off and on for about a year now, and I'd like to have menopause once and for all because, among other things, I have a strange metallic taste in my mouth that my doctor says is a menopausal symptom. Is that normal?"

Odd taste perceptions are a typical menopausal symptom, with "salty" and "metallic" the flavors women mention most often. They gradually disappear, but if you want to hurry their demise, take estrogen replacement when you finally reach menopause.

EVERYBODY'S DIFFERENT

If you are having unbearable menopausal symptoms and your next-door neighbor is saying, "I'm having no trouble at all. What's all the fuss about?" it does not mean you are a neurotic or she a better person. Nor does it mean that it's your fault or you've lived your life wrong. All it means is that every woman's body is different.

First, the number of estrogen receptors in the brain's hypothalamus is remarkably variable among perfectly normal women. Some women have 100,000 receptors clamoring to be supplied with estrogen, while others have only 2,000. When estrogen production shuts down, women with more receptors find themselves with the worst symptoms because they produce the highest levels of FSH, the pituitary hormone that sets off the vasomotor responses.

The severity of your symptoms is also a matter of the inherited rate at which you stop producing estrogen. If you are lucky enough to have hormone production that diminishes very slowly, your symptoms may hardly be noticeable. But if you lose estrogen rapidly, you will probably experience more uncomfortable effects. That's why women who lose their hormone supply abruptly because of surgery or ovarian damage from illness, radiation, or chemotherapy usually have the worst symptoms of all.

"Do overweight women tend to have especially bad hot flashes?"

Sometimes yes, sometimes no. Their greater skin surface and stressed circulation makes them more susceptible to the disruptions in heat regulation that lead to hot flashes. On the other hand, menopause is sometimes easier for overweight women because the fat cells convert other sex hormones manufactured in the ovaries and adrenal glands into estrogen, even after menopause. In some overweight women, that additional estrogen is enough to fend off severe flashes.

"I have a terrible time sleeping these days. I don't fall asleep at night for at least an hour, sometimes more, after I get into bed. How is this connected with menopause?"

Insomnia is a common menopausal complaint, and it is probably the second most common reason (hot flashes are number one) why women seek help from their doctors at this time. There are two reasons why you are likely to be suffering from sleep disturbances now.

If you are having episodes of hot flashes and drenching sweats during the night, you are certainly not going to get a good night's sleep. But even more important, *sleep latency increase* is a classic menopausal symptom. *Sleep latency* is professional jargon for the time that elapses between closing your eyes and falling asleep. For some women that time becomes longer and longer after menopause if they don't take estrogen. The same hypothalamic disturbances that cause hot flashes also produce a change in brain waves that produces insomnia—both sleep latency and wakeful periods during the night. That's because the hypothalamus controls sleep as well as temperature and hormone production.

To compound the problem, women with an estrogen deficiency tend not to sleep as soundly as they used to, spending less time in deep REM sleep and more time in light and fitful sleep.

"What usually triggers hot flashes? I get them whenever I drink coffee."

Almost anything can trigger hot flashes in susceptible women, especially if its usual effect is to raise body temperature or dilate the capillaries in the skin. Hot drinks, exercise, excitement, anxiety, stress, and excessive clothing all tend to raise your temperature, while alcohol, caffeine, and spicy foods cause the capillaries to dilate.

"How come I'm now having hot flashes even though I had a hysterectomy more than ten years ago? I am now 56."

A hysterectomy, by definition, is the surgical removal of the uterus. It does not necessarily include removal of the ovaries (an oophorectomy). It's surprising how many women have no idea whether or not they still have their ovaries. Obviously, you have yours. So, even though you had no menstrual periods after your operation, you were still producing estrogen. Now your ovaries are closing up shop and you are having menopause along with its symptoms.

"I can tolerate the hot flashes but I don't like feeling jumpy, irritable, and tense all the time. What's going on?"

Menopause definitely has an emotional component. During this time when hormone levels are changing, it is not uncommon for women to feel edgy and emotionally fragile, perhaps with mood swings much like PMS. That's because a shift in the level of any sex-related hormone can affect mood, and estrogen is no exception. Tension is a symptom that occurs most often and most severely in women whose hormone supply is abruptly or rapidly ended. On the other hand, it is usually an early symptom and almost always goes away within a year.

"Is there any truth to the old wives' tale that menopause can make women go crazy?"

None whatsoever, although women who already have emotional problems may find them accentuated by fluctuating hormone levels and disrupted sleep patterns.

"I find I'm forgetting things more and more these days. I've heard this happens at menopause. What can be done about it?"

Many women complain that their memory is impaired right after menopause, especially their recall of names of things or people. Unfortunately, hormone replacement doesn't seem to help and nobody knows what does.

"I've developed dry eyes since I had menopause. Is there a connection?"

A lack of circulating estrogen decreases the fluid output in many parts of the body, including the eyes, nose, and mouth. Dry eyes are common after menopause, most noticeably in women who had previously produced a low level of secretions. Artificial tears, in over-the-counter preparations, will help and so will hormone replacement, often quite dramatically. Always report your dry eyes to your doctor, however, because several disorders can cause them, too.

WHAT TO DO ABOUT SYMPTOMS

Menopausal symptoms aren't life-threatening and they will fade away in time, but that doesn't mean you have to live with them if they are adversely affecting the quality of your life. You can take hormone replacement therapy, which will turn all of these symptoms into a memory within a week or two. For eight out of ten women, two years of hormone replacement—daily or cyclical estrogen supplements plus progesterone supplements to protect the uterus—are sufficient for weathering the symptoms.

But if for medical reasons you can't, or for other reasons you don't wish to, take estrogen, there are several alternative methods that may provide some relief. None of them, however, is anywhere near as effective as HRT.

Progesterone Therapy   For women who can't take estrogen, the next best medical choice is small daily doses of oral progesterone. Though certainly not as helpful as estrogen, this second most important female hormone sometimes works well enough to get you through the worst of your symptomatic phase.

Other Alternative Drugs   A few medications can diminish, although seldom eliminate, vasomotor episodes and may be helpful when intervention is badly needed but estrogen therapy is out of the question. They include clonidine (Catapres), which is commonly used for hypertension and may lower normal blood pressure too much; and Bellergal, an antispasmodic drug with some notable side effects that include slowdown of digestion and blurred vision.

Vitamin E   Nobody knows why, but this vitamin frequently helps women with mild symptoms. Because it is impossible to get an effective dose of vitamin E from food (good sources are wheat germ, whole grains, nuts, safflower oil), you must take it in supplements. Start with 400 units twice a day for a total of 800 units. If that doesn't do it within a week or so, double the dose for a total of 1,600 units a day. (Caution: In rare instances in susceptible people, large doses of vitamin E have been found to raise blood pressure.)

Vitamins B and C There are no scientific studies to prove the effectiveness of these vitamins, but there has been considerable testimony that vitamins B and C can be helpful in relieving symptoms including depression, tension, and distressful mood swings. Start with one B-50 tablet, 400 to 500 milligrams of vitamin B_6, and 500 milligrams of vitamin C once a day.

Tranquilizers and Antidepressants Tranquilizers like Valium and antidepressants like Prozac are often prescribed for menopausal symptoms. The problem is that both tranquilizers and antidepressants can be habit-forming with severe withdrawal symptoms, so use them carefully and infrequently and make them a distant second choice to hormone therapy.

Natural Remedies Herbs and roots have been used for centuries for the treatment of "female complaints," and if they work for you, that's fine. Some women swear by such natural remedies as ginseng, dong quai, wild yam, evening primrose oil, soybeans, and sage for menopausal symptoms. To tell the truth, they may be quite effective, although the medical community in general does not recommend them. Some of these remedies, called phytoestrogens, are potent sources of natural plant estrogen and therefore are actually a form of estrogen-replacement therapy.

Small doses of these natural substances probably won't hurt you and may do you some good, but prolonged use, especially in large amounts, is just like taking estrogen without the opposing progesterone. It can result in hyperplasia—an overproliferation of the uterine lining—that, unless diagnosed and treated, can lead to cancer.

Pro-gest, another "natural" remedy that contains progesterone synthesized from Mexican yams, has become very popular as a treatment for all kinds of female complaints, including menopausal symptoms. A cream applied topically to the abdomen and buttocks, it is absorbed through the skin. Some women claim it is very helpful, but like many other natural remedies, it has not been scientifically tested and nobody knows how much vegetable progesterone it may deliver into the bloodstream. An overdose of any drug, whatever its source, is never a good idea.

Always take herbs and roots in moderation, remembering that some can cause allergic reactions, some have surprising side effects such as high blood pressure and palpitations, and others are toxic in large quantities. Buy your herbs in a reputable store because they are available in many varieties and grades. Consult an experienced herbalist for the proper dosage.

Increased Consumption of Fruits and Vegetables Eat more plant foods and cut back on animal products and you may find your symptoms alleviated, according to nutritionist Carol Devine of Cornell University. Japanese women who eat mostly fruits and vegetables and Western women who are vegetarians excrete significantly higher levels of estrogen in their urine and often suffer less from symptoms. Plant estrogens are found in many plant foods from apples to alfalfa sprouts to split peas, spinach, and especially soybean products and linseed.

Acupuncture, Biofeedback, and Relaxation Techniques Although there are no scientific studies to back up the testimonial evidence that these methods can relieve vasomotor menopausal symptoms, some women report that they offer considerable relief. Acupuncture and biofeedback are currently under study. Relaxation techniques including meditation have been found to ease many kinds of discomforts and will certainly help you cope with the stress and tension they may cause.

Deep Breathing A recent study found that slow, deep, abdominal breathing—six to eight times a minute—can reduce the occurrence of hot flashes for some women. Do your breathing for about ten minutes morning and night.

Exercise Physical activity may alleviate the symptoms, according to a recent study. Researchers at the University of Illinois found that women who spent the most time engaged in such activities as dancing or tennis reported experiencing fewer hot flashes and night sweats, fewer mood swings, fewer problems with urinary incontinence and vaginal dryness. Their general health was better, too.

Other Sensible Solutions Turn on the air-conditioning, take frequent cool showers, sip cold drinks, dress in removable layers, wear absorbent materials, get enough rest and exercise, try to avoid stress, and eat an adequate balanced diet. Cut out the triggers, such as alcohol and caffeine, that may set off hot flashes.

We'll Say It Once More!

Needless suffering won't get you into heaven, and there is no reason to spend valuable time with menopausal symptoms that make you miserable. If you have tried all of the alternative measures described here and have found none that works for you, break down and take HRT at least for the short term (unless, of course, it is medically contraindicated in your case). Taking hormones under a qualified doctor's supervision, if only for the year or two it takes for the symptoms to subside, is not only safe but sane.

Although some physicians are concerned about the possible side effects of taking hormones, there are no known problems with short-term estrogen. All of the

current controversy involves long-term HRT—hormones taken for ten years or more. However, virtually
all of the top experts agree that even a lifetime of taking
replacement hormones is safe for the vast majority of
women.

THE UNIVERSAL CHANGES

The typical temporary menopausal symptoms are the most
obvious effects of the monumental adjustment your body
makes to a new level of estrogen. But they don't happen to
the same degree for every woman, and they are by no means
the most important aspect of estrogen deficiency.

Much more significant to your health, comfort, and future
well-being is the fact that many tissues throughout the body
have receptors for estrogen, meaning that the hormone stimulates them in some way. Without the influence of estrogen,
they respond by making changes too, all of them of an atrophic
nature. These changes can be the cause of new discomforts
and conditions that can last indefinitely and almost always
get worse over time.

Every woman's timetable for these universal physical
changes is different. If your estrogen production diminishes
slowly and your ovaries and fat tissue continue to produce
some estrogen after menopause, the atrophic changes will
occur at a more leisurely pace. But if it happens quickly,
especially as the result of having your ovaries removed or
suppressed, they will come about much more rapidly.

Here's what is going on:

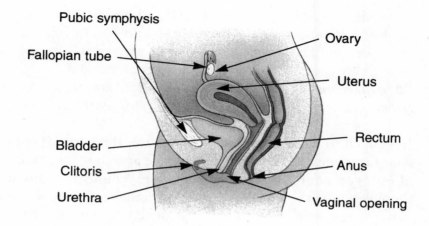

- Your ovaries and uterus, no longer needed for conception and pregnancy, shrink to about a third their former size.
- The endometrium—the lining of the uterus—thins and finally becomes nonfunctioning.
- The flow of mucus from the cervix and vagina gradually diminishes.
- The vagina and vulva shrink and the vaginal walls become thinner, drier, more fragile, less resilient, less lubricated (see Chapter 11).
- The urethra's tissues become thinner and more easily damaged. The distance between the vagina and the urethra grows shorter (see Chapter 15).
- The bladder loses muscle tone and elasticity, becomes less able to hold urine (see Chapter 16).
- The muscles that form the pelvic floor and support your internal organs become more lax.
- The breasts lose their formerly thick layer of fat and the milk glands shrink (see Chapter 6).
- The skin loses much of its underlying layer of fat and becomes thinner, drier, and more lax (see Chapter 18).
- The bones start to lose mass at an accelerated rate, becoming more porous and fragile (see Chapter 4).
- The cardiovascular system loses the beneficial effect of estrogen on HDL cholesterol—the kind that protects

against heart disease—and LDL, the kind that contributes to plaque in the arteries. The arteries become narrower and less elastic (see Chapter 5).

"Are there any advantages to having a late menopause? My friend had hers at 39, but I'm 57 and still waiting."

In general, the later you have menopause, the better it is for your future health. The longer you have an abundant amount of estrogen nourishing your tissues, the "younger" many of them will remain. The only real disadvantage of a late menopause is a very slight increase in the incidence of breast cancer and a slightly higher risk of ovarian cancer.

"I have to get up two or three times a night to urinate. Is that a menopausal symptom? If not, what's the reason for it?"

It's a result of both aging and menopause. Without abundant estrogen to maintain the muscle tone and elasticity of the bladder, its capacity to hold urine is smaller. So you feel the urge to go with less fluid content than before. The trips to the bathroom during the night may also be connected with menopause in another way: you are probably not sleeping as well as you used to (a menopausal symptom) and a full bladder wakes you up more easily.

THE BENEFITS OF HORMONE REPLACEMENT THERAPY

Hormone replacement therapy (HRT) cannot keep the effects of aging and estrogen deprivation at bay indefinitely after your ovaries go out of business. But it can make a tremendous difference in many ways by retarding some of the changes in estrogen-dependent tissues, sometimes even reversing them. That's because:

- *Bones.* HRT is the *only* effective way to stop bone loss and prevent osteoporosis after menopause. Women who take HRT sustain 40 percent fewer hip fractures than those who don't take it (see Chapter 4).
- *Heart.* Although estrogen has not yet been approved by the FDA specifically for the prevention of heart disease, many important studies have shown that HRT protects women against cardiovascular disease. On average, women on HRT live significantly longer than other women, suffer 44 percent fewer heart attacks, and have cut their risk of heart disease almost in half (see Chapter 5).

   This protection is thought to be the result of estrogen's ability to raise the levels of HDL cholesterol—the "good" cholesterol that helps keep the artery walls clear of plaque—while lowering LDL—the harmful cholesterol. In fact, most specialists in the field agree that estrogen has a more profound effect in altering the HDL-LDL ratio than any cholesterol-lowering drug currently available. According to one big study, taking estrogen plus progesterone reduces by half the level of a form of LDL called Lp(a) that increases risk for blocked arteries. Estrogen may also have a direct beneficial effect on the elasticity of the arterial walls themselves and may decrease the incidence of stroke. It also increases blood flow and dilates arteries.
- *Vagina.* HRT helps restore the lining, shape, and secretions of the vagina to its former elastic, lubricated state, thereby eliminating the problem of painful sex (see Chapter 7).
- *Urethra.* HRT restores the tissues of the urethra, preventing recurring urinary infections. It also improves the elasticity of the bladder (see Chapter 15).
- *Body.* HRT helps maintain the firmness and strength of muscle tissue as well as keep skin younger, breasts firmer, hair stronger (see Chapter 18).

- *Pain.* It can dramatically relieve muscle pain as well as the joint pains that tend to start with menopause.
- *Alzheimer's Disease.* HRT may reduce the chances of getting Alzheimer's disease and, if you do get it, may result in milder symptoms.
- *Mood.* Estrogen replacement improves mood, reduces stress, and enhances a sense of well-being.

"Is it true that estrogen replacement is dangerous? I don't like taking drugs of any kind and I'd rather not take estrogen either. I've read that it can cause cancer."

If you need the benefits of estrogen after menopause, you should certainly take it and stop worrying about it. Estrogen replacement is absolutely safe when used *correctly*, which means in low doses, combined with the hormone progesterone, individually prescribed, and monitored regularly. Not only will it *not* give you cancer but it will help protect you *against* it. The incidence of uterine cancer among women on HRT (a combination of estrogen and progesterone) has been found to be significantly *lower* than among those not on it.

As for the possibility of an increased risk of breast cancer, the results are not all in. Some studies have shown a slightly increased risk, others a slightly decreased risk, while still others no effect at all. What is clear is that in the average healthy woman, low-dose estrogen-only replacement therapy for fifteen years does not increase the risk of breast cancer. The modern combined estrogen-progesterone HRT has not been used long enough to evaluate its effects on breast cancer, but all data suggest that the effects will be small one way or the other.

Estrogen is not a carcinogen and does not initiate cancer, although it can accelerate the growth of a cancer that is already present. The good news is that, according to one very large study, when a woman on HRT develops an early breast cancer, her prognosis is much better than it is for a woman who takes no hormones. Perhaps this is because estrogen makes the cancer grow more rapidly but not more malignantly, and it can be picked up at a still curable stage.

HRT also protects against osteoporosis, which can be disabling and life-threatening, and coronary heart disease, the number one disabler and killer of them all.

To sum it up, women who use hormone replacement therapy live significantly longer than those who don't.

"Would you recommend HRT to most women today?"

Yes, if there are no specific contraindications to its use. Medical opinion is unanimous that the benefits of HRT far outweigh the risks. With very few exceptions, every woman can safely take HRT at least on a short-term basis, which means anywhere from a few months to five years. The vast majority of women should seriously consider it.

"How long can I stay on HRT?"

Forever, if you are monitored regularly by your gynecologist (as every woman should be with or without HRT). Many women need estrogen for ten or more years or perhaps for the rest of their lives, especially if they are at high risk for osteoporosis or heart disease. Others need it to preserve their sex lives and prevent recurring urinary problems. It is safe and beneficial to take it for a lifetime if you remember the guidelines: low doses, progesterone if you have a uterus, checkups every six months, mammograms once a year.

"How many women in the United States currently take estrogen? And how many stay on it?"

Fewer than 15 percent of postmenopausal American women who could benefit from estrogen replacement are actually taking it. About 20 percent stop taking it within nine months and another 20 to 30 percent get a prescription for it but never have it filled. Some are afraid of cancer; others don't like having periods (which can be avoided) or have uncomfortable side effects (which can usually be eliminated). We have found in our own practices, however, that women rarely drop out on their own when they have had HRT carefully explained to them and/or their dosages or schedules have been adjusted to alleviate the "nuisance" side effects.

"I don't like taking drugs and I want to take hormones only as long as I really need them. How long should I stay on them?"

If you are interested only in relieving menopausal symptoms such as hot flashes and insomnia, then two to five years should be enough. If, after gradually withdrawing from estrogen, the symptoms don't come back, fine, you don't need it anymore.

If, however, you are most interested in preventing osteoporosis, you should stay on HRT for at least ten years after menopause to get you through the time when bone loss is most severe.

If you look and feel wonderful on HRT, and have no bothersome side effects, you can stay on forever. After all, it protects your bones and your heart as well as your vagina and your urinary tract and it doesn't cause cancer. Besides, you don't have to decide *now* how long you'll stay on it. Wait for your next annual gynecological checkup to decide how you feel about it and what you want to do.

"We all worry about Alzheimer's disease these days when we've lost our car keys or can't remember what we were looking for in the closet. Is it really true that taking estrogen after menopause reduces the chances of developing it?"

At a recent scientific meeting, researchers from the University of Southern California in Los Angeles presented credible evidence that women who take estrogen appear to have less chance of getting Alzheimer's, and when they do get it, have milder symptoms. The hormone appears to help preserve brain cells involved in learning and memory. In a study of 253 women over several years, it was found that 18 percent of those who had not had estrogen were diagnosed with the disease, compared to 7 percent of those who had the therapy after menopause. Not only that, but the women who took the hormone but still got Alzheimer's performed better than average on cognitive tests.

In another study, scientists studied 8,879 women in retirement communities for information on their medical histories. They then reviewed the death certificates for the 2,418 women who died from 1981 to 1992 to find out which ones had Alzheimer's. They found that women on estrogen replacement were 40 percent less likely to have the disease or related dementias, compared to women who had not taken the hormone.

By the way, Alzheimer's is three times more common in women than men.

"I read recently that women who take estrogen after menopause are smarter than those who don't. Is there any truth to that?"

According to new research reported at a meeting of the American College of Neuropsychopharmacology, estrogen is a cognitive enhancer, and there is "clear and significant" improvement in mental ability from the hormone. A small group of women tested before and after they started HRT showed improvement in scores in tests that measured memory, eye-hand coordination, reflexes, and the ability to learn and apply new information.

HRT: THE SIDE EFFECTS

Usually, the side effects of hormone replacement therapy are nuisance effects, minor and transient. But occasionally they are uncomfortable enough to consider giving up the hormones. Most of these effects are caused by the progesterone you must take given along with the estrogen to protect the lining of your uterus, if you still have one. If you quit taking progesterone because of its side effects, however, you *must* have an annual endometrial biopsy or examination by vaginal probe ultrasound to make certain your uterine lining is not growing too rapidly.

Here is a rundown of the most usual side effects of taking HRT:

Monthly Periods Estrogen has the job of thickening the endometrium while progesterone's role is to precipitate the shedding of that thickened uterine lining. For at least a few years after you start HRT (if you take the progesterone for only part of the month), you will have a brief light menstrual response or period every month. If you find the periods objectionable, ask your gynecologist about switching to continuous progesterone. This means taking the progesterone in very low doses *every* day of the month. By the fourth month on this regime, eight out of every ten women have no more periods except perhaps for intermittent spotting.

Fluid Retention Most women notice some fluid retention, if only for the first few weeks after starting hormone treatment. This is not a serious complication and it usually goes away before long, but you might cut down on your salt intake and take vitamin B_6, a natural diuretic, in doses of 500 milligrams a day.

If the bloating is major, doesn't disappear on its own, and vitamin B_6 doesn't help enough, you might try a diuretic. Aldactone (spironolactone), available by prescription, is the diuretic of choice because it is very mild and may be taken every day if necessary.

Breast Tenderness This side effect usually is only a temporary problem and dissipates after three or four months.

Meanwhile, you can ease your discomfort with an over-the-counter pain reliever. Some women do best when they take their estrogen cyclically—three weeks on, one week off—rather than continuously. If the discomfort continues, perhaps your doctor will see if a different type of progesterone (a 19 nor-steroid, for example) eliminates the problem. Or you might try taking your progesterone in low doses every day of the month. Another option is to take estrogen combined with a tiny dose of testosterone, the male hormone that every woman produces in her ovaries and adrenal glands.

Weight Gain   Many women gain two or three pounds when they start HRT, probably because of fluid retention—a situation some don't mind but others find very hard to live with. Don't blame your hormones, however, for a major weight gain. That's more likely to be caused by the natural tendency of all of us to put on new pounds in new places as we get older.

Headaches   Sometimes women, especially those who tend to get migraines, complain that hormone supplements give them headaches. Often this problem can be solved by taking the smallest possible dose of estrogen, or by changing the type of estrogen, switching to the estrogen patch instead of oral pills, or taking estrogen combined with a tiny dose of testosterone.

If the headaches are found to be due to the progesterone and you need estrogen badly, you can quit the progesterone but *only* if you have no unexpected bleeding *and* have an endometrial biopsy or ultrasound measurement of the endometrium once a year.

Nausea   This is the most common side effect of HRT taken orally, but it usually wears off before long. If it doesn't, switch to the transdermal patch, which gives you estrogen directly through the skin rather than through the digestive system.

Allergy   There is the occasional woman who has typical allergic responses—rashes, swelling, itching—to HRT. If you are that woman, try a different type of estrogen or progesterone, try taking estrogen by patch, or wait and see if you adjust to it.

PMS-like Symptoms   Some women find that progesterone makes them feel irritable, jumpy, tense, or depressed, much like PMS. Usually these feelings vanish after a while along with the fluid retention. But if they don't dissipate after a couple of months on cyclical progesterone, talk to your doctor about taking a slightly increased dose of estrogen on the days that overlap your cyclical progesterone.

An alternative is to discontinue the cyclical schedule and take your progesterone in the everyday continuous low-dose way described later in this chapter. The smaller dose may not give you those PMS-like symptoms.

A more dramatic alternative, if you really need estrogen but can't tolerate progesterone's effect, is to stop the progesterone and take estrogen alone. Never do this on your own but always under your doctor's supervision. If you have not had your uterus removed, you must be sure your endometrium does not become dangerously thickened by the estrogen. This means yearly surveillance by endometrial biopsy or ultrasound measurements of the endometrium.

Skin Reactions   Sometimes the transdermal estrogen patch causes redness, irritation, or itching at the site where it is placed. Usually this problem dissipates after a few weeks. Make sure you apply the patch to clean dry skin and, after air-drying it for about five seconds, try wearing it on the buttocks, where the skin is usually less sensitive than the abdomen.

Drug Sensitivity   For supersensitive women, oral estrogen heightens the sensitivity to some drugs also cleared by the liver. The solution is to switch to the transdermal patch, which delivers estrogen directly into the bloodstream through the skin, thereby missing the first pass through the liver.

CHOICES OF THERAPY

Currently there are three ways to take estrogen replacement: pills, patch, or vaginal cream. Progesterone is available by pill or suppository. Like any other drug, hormones should not be taken casually. They must be prescribed specifically for you and then monitored, and they should be taken in the smallest amounts that will accomplish their purpose. See the tables below for a list of common hormone preparations.

Commonly Used Estrogens and Progesterones

TRADE NAME	FORMS	MANUFACTURER
Premarin	tablets, vaginal cream	Wyeth-Ayerst
Generics	tablets	various
Ogen	tablets	Abbott
Estrace	tablets, vaginal cream	Mead Johnson
Estratabs	tablets	Solvay
Ortho-est	tablets	Ortho
Estraderm	skin patch	Ciba-Geigy
Dienestrol	vaginal cream	Ortho
Provera	tablets	Upjohn
Megace	tablets	Bristol-Myers
Norlutate	tablets	Parke-Davis
Aygestin	tablets	Wyeth-Ayerst
Utrogestin	tablets	to order
Progesterone	suppositories	to order

ORAL ESTROGEN

Most women on HRT take their estrogen by pill: one every day or one a day for the first twenty-five days of the month. The most widely prescribed form is conjugated estrogen (Premarin), a combination of natural estrogens and the subject of more than fifty years of scientific testing. Another that is rapidly becoming popular is Estrace (micronized estradiol), the closest equivalent of human estrogen.

A minimum dose of 0.625 milligrams (or its equivalent) is usually required to prevent the bone loss that becomes osteoporosis, and that's the dose most doctors will start you off with. However, the circulating estrogen level is more important than the dose, and some women may need as little as 0.3 milligrams or equivalent, while some need more than the standard dose. If you have a uterus, you must take progesterone too, every day of the month or overlapping your estrogen for ten to fourteen days a month.

In general, if you are under 40 when you have menopause, you'll require more estrogen than if you stop menstruating at the usual age. You may have to start with 0.9 milligrams, still considered a low dose, or perhaps 1.25 milligrams, and then taper off later. And if you are suffering from serious vaginal atrophy, you may well need 2.5 milligrams a day, at least at the beginning.

Oral estrogen is usually taken once a day, but if you are having extremely severe symptoms, you may do better taking it in divided doses, half in the morning and half at night, to allow a more even blood level throughout the twenty-four hours.

We strongly recommend taking your estrogen every day because that follows the natural pattern more closely than taking it for three weeks and then skipping a week. The cyclical schedule was inherited from the one designed for oral contraceptives, which allowed for a menstrual period. But it's not necessary or even desirable to take a week off from HRT. Some women even get menopausal symptoms during that week. The only women who might want to stay on the old-fashioned schedule are those who find that a cyclical pattern gives them relief from persistent breast tenderness.

Estrogen by pill can sometimes aggravate such medical conditions as gallbladder disease, liver dysfunction, renin-hypertension, and thrombophlebitis. If this is the case for you, switch to the transdermal patch, which gives you estrogen unaltered by the digestive system.

TRANSDERMAL ESTROGEN PATCH

An alternative way to take estrogen, the patch delivers the hormone at a relatively constant rate directly into the blood-stream through the skin, making it the estrogen of choice if you have the medical problems mentioned above. When the hormone does not pass through the digestive system and the liver, it does not cause the release of enzymes that could adversely affect those conditions.

The patch comes in two varieties. Both are applied to clean dry skin on the abdomen or buttocks, changed twice a week, and are meant to be worn every day of the month. The first is Estraderm, a patch that looks much like a large round or oval Band-Aid and delivers the estrogen from a reservoir in its center. It is available in two dosages: 0.05 milligram (round) and 0.1 milligram (oval). The 0.05 milligram patch, the usual option, is the equivalent of somewhere between 0.3 milligram and 0.625 milligram of conjugated estrogen; while the 0.10 milligram patch is equivalent to between 0.9 and 1.25 milligrams of conjugated estrogen.

The newest generation of transdermal patch, at this writing unnamed and subject to FDA approval, uses a different method of delivering the estrogen. It is a matrix patch with the hormone embedded in the adhesive so that it is much smaller, thinner, more flexible, and more transparent than Estraderm. It is available in four dosages: 0.0375 milligram, 0.05 milligram, 0.075 milligram, and 0.01 milligram.

The patch is just as effective as the pill in reducing meno-pausal symptoms, reversing vaginal and urinary changes, and preventing osteoporosis. It also increases your level of HDL, the "good cholesterol" (although it takes a few months after you begin taking it before the effect can be seen).

You must take progesterone when you take estrogen by patch (unless you have had a hysterectomy or have a very poor reaction to this hormone), either every day or for your prescribed number of days each month.

VAGINAL ESTROGEN CREAM

Although estrogen cream inserted into the vagina is minimally absorbed into the bloodstream and affects other parts of the body, its main effect is on the tissues of the vagina and ure-thra. Except in special circumstances, it should not be consid-ered equivalent to estrogen taken by pill or transdermal patch. It reverses the vaginal and urethral changes caused by estro-gen deficiency, and it may help to alleviate mild symptoms, but it cannot be counted on to prevent osteoporosis or heart disease or to relieve severe hot flashes. For long-term hor-mone therapy, it's best to take your estrogen by pill or patch. With vaginal cream, it is almost impossible to know just how much of the hormone is being absorbed into the general circu-lation. And taking your estrogen by cream doesn't mean that you can forget about taking progesterone as well.

The cream is inserted into the vagina with a measured applicator. Doses must be individualized because absorption from vaginal cream varies from woman to woman, but 1 gram two or three times a week is usually sufficient. You and your doctor will have to work out a schedule and a dose that works for you. Most of the time, you will start off with a fairly high dose and then taper off after your tissues have returned to normal.

A benefit of estrogen taken vaginally is that, like transder-mal estrogen, it is not absorbed through the digestive system and so it is safe for women with medical conditions such as gallbladder disease and thrombophlebitis.

For more details about the vaginal cream and its effect on genital and urinary health as well as your sex life, see Chapters 7, 11, and 15.

EQUIVALENT ESTROGEN DOSES

How much estrogen do you need? The standard dose is 0.625 mg of Premarin or its equivalent. In most cases this is enough to banish hot flashes and other symptoms and ward off osteoporosis and heart disease. But you and your doctor must decide on the dose and the kind of estrogen that works best for you. The equivalents of 0.625 mg of oral conjugated estrogen (Premarin) are:

Ogen	0.625 mg
Estrace	1 mg
Estratabs	0.625 mg
Ortho-est	0.625 mg
Estraderm	0.05 mg

PROGESTERONE

The other female hormone that must be taken with estrogen to protect the uterus from cancer, progesterone is usually prescribed in doses of 5 or 10 milligrams (or the equivalent) for ten to fourteen days of the month. However, this schedule has a couple of drawbacks.

First, you will probably have a brief menstrual response each month starting a day or so after you stop taking the hormone, at least for the initial few years. Although the periods are abbreviated and light, most women dislike them. In fact, they are a major reason why many women abandon HRT.

Second, cyclical progesterone may cause PMS-like symptoms each month before the brief period.

The newest way to take progesterone is in very low doses—2.5 milligrams—every day of the month along with daily estrogen. This schedule eliminates the monthly menstrual response for about eight out of ten women after the first two or three months.

It does not, by the way, counteract estrogen's ability to raise HDL, the healthful blood lipids, and lower LDL, or to preserve bone mass.

"But I've read many times that estrogen can give you cancer of the uterus."

Estrogen itself is not a carcinogen and so it does not cause cancer. However, when it is not taken with progesterone, it can cause endometrial hyperplasia, an overgrowth of the cells that line the uterus. Hyperplasia is not cancer, but it may be a precancerous condition. Left untreated, it can set the stage for cancer in certain susceptible women.

Progesterone, the hormone that triggers the shedding of the thickened lining, must be taken along with estrogen if you are still in possession of your uterus. When enough progesterone is given each month in combination with a minimal amount of estrogen, there is no excessive buildup of tissue that could lead to cancer. In fact, when you take both hormones, you are *less* likely to develop cancer of the uterus than women who have never taken them.

"Are there any disadvantages to the transdermal estrogen patch?"

The only apparent side effect is occasional skin irritation caused by the adhesive. This usually improves once you become accustomed to it. By the way, the effects of the patch won't be diminished if you pull the patch off and reapply it to a different spot when it becomes bothersome.

And sometimes the patch comes off when you're bathing or swimming. The water won't hurt it, so just put it back on again, or take it off while you shower or swim. Or apply a new one and stay on your same replacement schedule.

The patch is more expensive than estrogen pills.

"Now I can expect to have short monthly periods because of the progesterone in HRT. What about other bleeding? When should I be concerned about it?"

Always. The bleeding that occurs as a result of cyclical progesterone replacement is virtually the same every month, varying no more than one or two days and only slightly in the amount of flow. If *any* bleeding occurs at *any* time other than those usual few days, or if it is prolonged, clotted, or very heavy, it must be investigated. Bleeding that does not occur according to plan requires an evaluation by your gynecologist.

"Should I be concerned because, after three years on HRT, I've stopped having periods?"

No. It simply means you now have an inactive endometrium and there's no buildup of lining to clear out each month. However, just to be safe, you should continue to take the progesterone.

"I can't tolerate progesterone. It gives me awful headaches and makes me terribly depressed. But I have both osteoporosis and heart disease in my family so I definitely want to take estrogen. What can I do?"

Perhaps you can tolerate the progesterone in lower doses. Talk to your doctor about switching to a continuous schedule of progesterone—2.5 milligrams every day of the month— rather than bigger doses for fewer days.

If that doesn't work, you can stay on estrogen and stop the

progesterone, but only if you do it correctly and cautiously. Until very recently, no responsible gynecologist would prescribe estrogen alone for a woman who still had her uterus because progesterone is the female hormone that protects the uterine lining from becoming overproliferated. But we've discovered that you can safely take estrogen alone *if* you and your doctor are willing to follow certain rigid rules.

First, there must be no "breakthrough" or unexpected vaginal bleeding. If you bleed on estrogen alone, that may mean the endometrium is being overstimulated.

Second, assuming you have no breakthrough bleeding, your uterine lining must be examined regularly—every six months at first, then if all is going well, every year. This is done by endometrial biopsy—a tiny piece of endometrial tissue is removed and examined under a microscope—or by vaginal ultrasound performed by an experienced technician.

Although abdominal ultrasound is sometimes used for this purpose, a vaginal ultrasound probe tends to be much more accurate. The ultrasound provides a way to measure the thickness of the uterine lining. If the endometrium is less than 6 mm thick, you have not developed hyperplasia, which always precedes endometrial cancer.

"Would you explain an endometrial biopsy? I had one about ten years ago and it was one of the worst experiences of my life."

That was then; this is now. An endometrial biopsy—removal of a small sample of cells from the lining of the uterus—is much less uncomfortable today because it is done with a very thin suction catheter instead of the big one used in the old days. Passed through the vagina and the opening of the cervix into the uterus, the pipelle removes sample cells in less than a minute. It can cause brief uterine cramps, however. If you find the cramping very uncomfortable, next time take two Advil tablets an hour before the procedure.

"What happens in a vaginal ultrasound probe?"

A tubular plastic instrument no larger than the speculum used for a pelvic examination, covered by a sterile disposable sheath or condom, is inserted in the vagina. Here, by means of sound waves, it sends back images of your ovaries and uterus, including the endometrium—all of which are viewed on a television monitor.

Keep Trying Until You Get It Right

Every woman's response to hormones is different, and not everyone responds immediately to the usual dosages, schedules, types of hormones, and routes of administration. But your doctor can individualize your treatment, trying alternatives until one is right for you. Be sure to alert the doctor promptly to any problems or questions you have. After all, the whole idea is that you will feel better on HRT.

"The reason I don't want to go on hormone replacement therapy is that I can't stand the idea of having periods again. Is there any way to avoid them?"

There are many women who truly dislike having even the short light periods that are part of the pattern for at least a few years when they take progesterone cyclically. This withdrawal bleeding that occurs just after you stop taking the progesterone each month is usually very light and very short, and eventually stops when the uterus becomes nonfunctioning.

But if you want to eliminate even these brief periods, try taking your progesterone in a continuous, everyday pattern. This means you take estrogen every day, by pill or patch, along with a low dose (2.5 milligrams) of medroxyprogester-one acetate (Provera) every day of the month. By the fourth month into this continuous regimen, which is just as safe as the cyclical schedule, 75 to 80 percent of women have no more periods.

Although most women stop having periods on the continuous method, some do continue to bleed irregularly. If the erratic spotting doesn't stop after about three months, you will probably need an endometrial biopsy to be sure that the uterine lining is not being overstimulated. If the lining is normal, you can safely continue taking the daily progesterone, although an annual ultrasound check of the endometrium is a good idea.

"If I've had a hysterectomy, do I have to take progesterone as well as estrogen?"

No. The purpose of including progesterone in HRT is solely to protect the uterus, and you no longer have one.

"I had a hysterectomy as a result of uterine cancer. Can I still take hormones?"

Yes, according to the newest thinking. A 1993 survey of members of the Society of Gynecologic Oncologists found that 83 percent of the responding cancer specialists approved of estrogen replacement for women who had had early stages of endometrial cancer, based on "prognostic indictators and the risk the patient was willing to assume." Formerly, the thinking was that estrogen should never be given to women who have had a uterine malignancy because, although it does not initiate cancer, it can accelerate the growth of cancer cells that are already there.

The Committee on Gynecologic Practice of the American College of Obstetricians and Gynecologists concluded: "For some women, the sense of well-being afforded by amelioration of menopausal symptoms or the need to treat atrophic vaginitis, provide cardiovascular protection, and reduce the risk of osteoporosis, may outweigh the risk of stimulating tumor growth."

"And what about all those reports of an increased risk of breast cancer?"

A panel of experts recently reviewed twenty-four studies of the possible connection between estrogen and breast cancer. The bottom line is that it is doubtful estrogen causes a higher risk of cancer. In our own study of a group of women who were followed for twenty-two years, we found there was no increase in the incidence of breast cancer among the women who took estrogen.

"Well, then, should every woman go on HRT?"

Every woman should consider it. If you can cope with the temporary menopausal symptoms without its help, that's fine. But when you review the benefits of HRT, especially regarding osteoporosis, heart disease, and sex life, it makes a pretty convincing argument.

"Does estrogen replacement affect the incidence of stroke in women?"

Strokes—the third leading cause of death in the United States—occur when an area of the brain is cut off from its arterial blood supply. They are caused by clots that block a significant artery or bleeding that disrupts the brain's function. Several recent studies have indicated that HRT can protect women against them. One study, for example, found that hormone use resulted in a 31 percent reduction in the incidence of stroke and in a 63 percent reduction in death caused by stroke.

WHO CAN'T TAKE HORMONES?

Today HRT is safe for virtually everyone except perhaps those women who have had estrogen-dependent breast cancer or advanced endometrial cancer, or who currently have acute active liver disease. Sometimes even in these cases, short-term estrogen is used to relieve severe vaginal or urinary atrophic problems. In fact, the most recent research shows no evidence that using estrogen increases the risk of developing new tumors among women who have already had breast cancer.

There are several other medical conditions that until recently ruled out HRT for many women who badly needed it. These included liver disorders, gallbladder disease, renin-hypertension, and thrombophlebitis. Some women on oral estrogen develop gallbladder problems because the hormone concentrates cholesterol in the bile. And a few women, about 8 percent, get an extra release of renin from the liver when they take estrogen by mouth, causing transient reversible hypertension.

But the transdermal estrogen patch and vaginal estrogen cream have made hormone therapy safe for virtually every woman in this group. When the hormone is delivered through the skin directly into the bloodstream, bypassing the digestive system on its first pass into the body, it has less effect on the liver. When estrogen cream is applied to the vagina in low doses, it is not readily absorbed into the bloodstream.

Even women who have had thrombophlebitis can take estrogen by patch without affecting their condition if, after a complete blood workup, it is found that they do not suffer from an abnormal blood-clotting disorder.

"I've had my gallbladder removed. Can I take estrogen?"

Certainly. Without a gallbladder, you no longer have to worry about gallstones or gallbladder disease, so feel free to take your estrogen by mouth if you like.

"My doctor took me off estrogen because my blood pressure went up, but I really need it for hot flashes. What can I do?"

Start taking your estrogen by transdermal patch, which doesn't have the same effect on the liver as estrogen taken orally and therefore does not precipitate higher blood pressure. About eight out of a hundred women have an extra release of renin from the liver that can cause a transient and reversible hypertension when they take oral estrogen.

"Is the estrogen in HRT as strong as the estrogen in birth-control pills?"

No, nowhere near as potent. The usual daily dose of 0.625 mg of conjugated estrogen is only about a third the amount used in the very lowest dose birth-control pills. Besides, the pill *adds* hormones to a menstruating woman's already normal hormone level. The hormones in HRT, given after menopause, *replace* those you no longer make for yourself.

"I have varicose veins. Is it true that I shouldn't take estrogen? I understand it can encourage blood clots."

Varicose veins are not a problem of clotting but, instead, of relaxed valves that allow the blood to pool and stretch the veins. The tiny amount of estrogen in HRT almost certainly won't make your veins worse, so we suggest you try it and see.

As for clotting, the low-dose estrogen used in HRT today has been found to have virtually no effect on the body's natural clot-fighting mechanisms—the anticlotting factors—

and then only in women who are supersensitive to it because of an abnormal blood condition. It is considered safe for everyone except perhaps women who have had serious clotting problems in the past. To find out if you are among them, have a complete medical evaluation of your anticlotting factors before you start taking estrogen if you have ever had thrombophlebitis (clots in deep veins), previous clotting problems during pregnancy or while on oral contraceptives, or a family history of such problems.

"I have rheumatoid arthritis and am debating whether to take hormones. I don't want to take any more drugs than I am already but I also need all the help I can get."

A recent study at the Multipurpose Arthritis Center at the University of California, San Francisco, reported that postmenopausal women with rheumatoid arthritis who are currently taking estrogen-replacement therapy experience milder arthritis symptoms than those who aren't. They have significantly fewer painful joints and better performance of daily activities.

Women, by the way, are two to three times more likely than men to have rheumatoid arthritis and often notice the first symptoms during perimenopause.

"Will HRT affect my fibrocystic breasts one way or another?"

There's no medical reason to avoid HRT just because you have fibrocystic breasts. Hormones do not make the condition worse, although they could make it more uncomfortable because of fluid retention. Try it and see.

"I've been told I can't take hormone replacement therapy because I have large fibroid tumors, but my mother and grandmother have osteoporosis. What should I do?"

Fibroids can be stimulated by high amounts of estrogen, but after menopause they usually shrink when hormone production drops. Furthermore, in most cases they continue to shrink even on hormone replacement because HRT gives you a smaller dose of estrogen than you used to make yourself. On the other hand, you should be checked every six months; if your fibroids do continue to grow, your physician may reduce your estrogen dosage or suggest you stop taking it.

Another way to go is to wait for a couple of years after menopause before starting to take hormones. Have your bone density measured and, if you are not at great risk for osteoporosis at the moment, hold off. The fibroids will usually shrink considerably during that time and you may then start HRT.

"My doctor hesitates to put me on hormone replacement even though I am having terrible symptoms because, he says, it could make my diabetes harder to control. What's your opinion?"

In our own ten-year study of a group of women on estrogen, we found that diabetic women had no negative effects from estrogen therapy. In fact, only two of twenty-six patients with diabetes experienced changes in their insulin requirements during that period of time. Because the estrogen dose is so low, it does not affect sugar metabolism. In any case, the diabetes can be managed properly while on HRT, although you may have to go through a short period of adjustment. We recommend, too, using the transdermal patch because diabetics have a higher-than-normal risk of gallbladder disease.

"Can I get pregnant when I'm taking hormone replacement?"

It is most unlikely but it is possible in early menopause. Just to be safe, use contraception for at least six months after your last period.

"I had my ovaries removed when I had a hysterectomy because of fibroids, and I have been having horrendous hot flashes, insomnia, and palpitations for six months. My doctor says I should live with them and they will go away eventually."

Women who have had their ovaries removed or damaged by radiation or chemotherapy usually have the most severe menopausal symptoms. Today it is a rare physician who will not prescribe estrogen at least for the short term, unless you have had estrogen-dependent cancer. Talk to your doctor again or find a doctor who is more sympathetic. There's absolutely no need to suffer.

"I've gained a lot of weight in the last few years, even though I'm not eating any differently. Can that be blamed on menopause?"

The blame probably lies mostly with a metabolic change that occurs somewhere around the age of 40, making it easier to gain weight with the same amount of food and exercise. In addition, most women have a tendency to gain a few pounds after menopause whether or not they take estrogen. This may have something to do with the fact that the female body, as it ages, gradually increases its ratio of fat to muscle. Fat tissue burns very few calories, so the older you are, the more exercise you need to stay the same (see Chapter 19).

What *does* change with menopause is your shape because your body is "feminized" by estrogen. With or without supplemental hormones, you tend to lose fat tissue in the hips and breasts, while the waist, shoulders, and upper back tend to become thicker. Meanwhile, your spine compresses, causing you to lose height and expand your rib cage (see Chapter 19).

"I have to urinate frequently, both day and night. Would estrogen replacement help me?"

Sometimes HRT has a really dramatic effect, sometimes not. Without estrogen, the bladder loses much of its elasticity. With estrogen replacement, some of that elasticity is restored. Perhaps even more important, HRT helps you get good, sound REM sleep. A sound sleeper isn't so likely to wake up several times during the night to go to the bathroom.

"When I had elective surgery recently, my doctor took me off estrogen two weeks before I went into the hospital. Why?"

In most cases, doctors recommend going off all nonessential medications before an operation to minimize the chance of drug interactions with medication you might be given in the hospital. Many doctors also remember the early years when high-dose birth-control pills caused problems with blood clotting, although that is not a problem with either the low-dose variety or HRT.

"Why do some doctors prescribe estrogen every day of the month while others give it to you cyclically for only three weeks of the month?"

Oral estrogen has traditionally been prescribed three weeks of the month with one week off simply because physicians have copied the schedule devised for birth-control pills, when a week off was required to allow for a menstrual period. But taking estrogen every day of the month is a much more accurate physiological pattern, providing a constant level of the hormone in the bloodstream. Most doctors are switching over to this pattern. Or they are prescribing the transdermal estrogen patch, which is worn every day and gives a consistent estrogen level.

Besides mimicking the normal premenopausal physiological pattern, taking estrogen every day has an advantage for women who suffer from vasomotor symptoms such as hot flashes on their "week off." With no interruption in the estrogen supply, the symptoms no longer make an unwelcome appearance every month.

On the other hand, if estrogen makes your breasts very tender, as it does for some women, you may do better with a week off once a month.

"What about the estrogen gel that women are using in Europe?"

The estrogen gel is not on the market in the United States yet, nor has it been approved by the FDA, but it looks promising. The gel is rubbed into the skin anywhere on the body once a day on an everyday or three-weeks-out-of-four pattern.

"And the vaginal ring?"

The vaginal ring is used in Sweden and is now being studied in the United States. Inserted in the vagina like a diaphragm and changed every twelve weeks, the ring releases a very tiny amount of estradiol, a pure form of estrogen, each day, relieving vaginal and urinary symptoms. The ring shows great promise especially for women whose sex lives are greatly affected by vaginal changes after menopause but who can't take estrogen systemically. The estrogen dose is so infinitesimal that it is not absorbed into the bloodstream.

"Is it ever too late for HRT? I had menopause more than ten years ago and now I want to take it, if it will do any good, because of poor bone-density measurements and extremely painful sex. Can hormones help me now?"

It's never too late. At any age, when you start taking estrogen, the continuous bone loss will stop, although the bone you have already lost cannot be significantly replaced. Unless you have waited far too long, HRT will rejuvenate your vaginal and urethral tissues, restore your ability to have comfortable intercourse, and make you more resistant to vaginal and urinary infections. It will give you some protection against cardiovascular disease by raising your HDL level.

"Do you lose all the benefits of HRT when you stop taking it?"

Yes, although in the meantime you have gained a few years of protection against bone loss and heart disease. And you have kept your vaginal and urethral tissues in good condition for that period of time as well.

"I've decided I don't want to take replacement hormones anymore. How should I quit?"

Never quit cold turkey or you may have menopausal symptoms all over again. You can best fool the estrogen receptors in your brain by tapering off very gradually, perhaps taking your estrogen every other day for a month, twice a week for another month, then once a week for a third month, all the while taking your usual amount of progesterone. If your hot flashes or other symptoms don't return, you can eventually quit altogether.

If you are stopping because of side effects, consider that a different combination of hormones may give you the benefits of HRT without any of the problems.

Chapter 4

YOUR BONES: WHEN YOU SHOULD WORRY ABOUT THEM

YOU SHOULD START THINKING about your bones *now*. The stronger they are before menopause, the stronger they will remain for the rest of your life. Bone mass reaches its peak density at about the age of 30. That's when you have as much bone as you're ever going to get. After that, bone tissue and strength begin to decline in everyone, man or woman. Lose enough of it, and you have significant osteoporosis.

Osteoporosis, the "disease of the decade," isn't a disease at all. Instead, it is a condition—part of the natural aging process—that is absolutely normal, natural, and universal. Everybody has it to one degree or another after the age of 40. What you have to be concerned about is that you don't allow it to develop to the point where it becomes symptomatic—in other words, where your bones become so fragile that they break easily.

WHAT YOU CAN DO *NOW*

Osteoporosis can't be cured, but it can be prevented. About half of your risk of developing it stems from not having enough bone to start with. So if you are premenopausal, start consuming enough calcium to attain the highest possible bone density by menopause, when you will lose bone tissue at an accelerated rate. In addition, be sure to get weight-bearing exercise a few times a week. Stop smoking. Drink only in moderation. Seriously consider hormone replacement therapy after menopause. Look into alternative treatments if you are at high risk and can't take estrogen.

OSTEOPOROSIS EXPLAINED

Osteoporosis is a fancy name for bones that have lost some of their mass, bulk, and density, making them subject to fracture. The most common bone disorder in the world, it starts slowly and silently—at a rate of about 1 percent a year—after the age of 30 or so. Then, with menopause, the loss accelerates to 2 to 3 percent a year, and in some cases as much as 10 percent, especially in the first seven years, before it drops back to about 1 percent again. Some illnesses, habits, and medications speed the loss even more.

But because there are no warning signs of serious bone loss, except perhaps mysterious backaches, you probably won't know you're about to have trouble until you have it, usually in the form of a fracture. Sometimes you won't even know it then, because some fractures—such as those in the spine—can occur without any pain. And by then, the disease is well under way. More than a million and a half Americans suffer fractures related to osteoporosis each year.

About Bones

Bones are living tissue that is constantly changing. The skeleton serves as a reservoir for calcium, storing it and releasing it when it is needed by other parts of the body. Through a process called *remodeling*, old bone tissue is continually being replaced with new, so the skeleton that's yours today is certainly not the one you'll have a few years from now.

Because osteoporosis is not significantly reversible and the lost bone can never be appreciably replaced, it is essential to prevent major bone depletion from occurring in the first place. Before menopause, there is usually a fairly good balance between the bone that is lost and the bone that replaces it—if you consume enough calcium. But after menopause, bone mass is lost much faster than it can be replaced, especially in the first six to eight years—no matter how much calcium you eat or how much exercise you get. So your bones gradually become more porous and fragile unless you take supplemental estrogen.

Calcium and exercise will help you retain some of the bone tissue, but the only way to put a complete halt to the process is to go on hormone replacement therapy for life because estrogen regulates the absorption of calcium. The experts agree today that hormone therapy *plus* sufficient calcium and exercise are the way to go for most women.

WHO GETS OSTEOPOROSIS? MEN VS. WOMEN

Everybody, male and female, can get osteoporosis. It affects more than 25 million people in the United States, 80 percent of them women.

It is normal for everyone's bones to become thinner and less dense as you get older. But, when it comes to bones, men are luckier than women. Men also lose bone with age, but since they start out with a heavier skeleton, it takes longer before they suffer the consequences. Besides, they do not have menopause. Their production of testosterone, the primary male hormone that regulates the absorption of calcium into the bones, doesn't drop off precipitously, as estrogen does in women. Instead, it declines gradually and, if men are going to develop breakable bones, it's usually not until they are very old. Finally, men don't live as long as women and they may not survive to an age when fractures become a major problem.

Women, who start out with a flimsier bone structure, can't afford to lose as much bone as men and so they are four times as likely to get symptomatic osteoporosis. According to the American Academy of Orthopedic Surgeons, women ultimately lose 30 to 50 percent of their bone density, while men lose 20 to 30 percent. Osteoporosis in the spine is eight times more prevalent among women than men, while the rate of hip fractures is two to three times higher in women than men.

And in 25 to 35 percent of women, bone loss after menopause becomes so extensive—especially in the spine, hip, and wrist—that it can result in life-threatening fractures.

ARE YOU A PRIME CANDIDATE FOR OSTEOPOROSIS?

You are in danger of developing symptomatic osteoporosis resulting in broken bones or compression of the spine by the time you are 65 or 70 (sometimes earlier) if you are:

• Thin
• Fair-skinned
• Small-boned
• A dieter and a milk hater

- An Asian or of northern European ancestry
- A consumer of more than two alcoholic drinks a day
- A smoker
- A woman with a sedentary lifestyle
- A woman who had an early menopause, natural or surgical
- A woman whose mother or grandmother has grown shorter over the years or who has had fractures
- A person who is a long-term user of steroid or thyroid drugs

Additional risk factors for osteoporosis include such chronic diseases as diabetes, rheumatoid arthritis, seizures, inflammatory bowel disease, hyperparathyroidism, and asthma, as well as illnesses or accidents that result in prolonged periods of immobilization.

NOT EVERYBODY'S IN DANGER

Not all women, of course, are in danger of developing seriously brittle bones. Some have such sturdy skeletons and superior muscle structure that they may never be seriously affected because they can lose considerable bone mass and still remain strong, even if they don't take estrogen after menopause. Others have a genetic resistance to osteoporosis. And overweight women may continue to make enough estrogen in their fat tissue long after menopause to help them absorb calcium.

But if you have a light frame, especially if you have inherited a gene that inhibits the absorption of calcium into the bone cells, and have not built up your bones with enough calcium and exercise during your peak years, you start off your middle years with a smaller margin of safety. And you must be especially careful to do whatever you can to prevent future problems.

FRACTURE FACTS

- Women over the age of 65 have a one-in-five chance of having a hip fracture during their lifetime. By age 80, about a third of all women in the United States have broken a hip because of osteoporosis, with one in five dying of complications within a year (hip fracture is, in fact, the most common cause of accidental death in women over the age of 75) and more than half of the survivors requiring extensive rehabilitation and long-term care. And as the American population continues to age, the number of hip fractures grows higher each year.

  In one study of 2,000 women, evidence of spinal osteoporosis was found in 29 percent of those between the ages of 45 and 54, 61 percent from 55 to 65, and 79 percent over 65.

- Often the first sign of the loss of spinal bone mass is back pain, or noticeably shorter stature, or the appearance of a "dowager's hump." The hump is caused by the collapse of spinal vertebrae when porous, brittle bones can no longer support the weight of the upper body. In fact, many of the aches and pains of older people result from tiny microfractures and spinal compressions they don't even know they have. As the bone loss continues, even a minor fall can result in the fracture of fragile bones, frequently ending in restricted mobility and chronic pain.

- Women with very low bone mass—in other words, significant osteoporosis—have a 40 percent chance of breaking a hip. Statistics show that a woman with average bone mass at menopause has only a 15 percent chance of suffering a hip fracture in her lifetime.

"How can I find out if my bones are in good shape? I am 47 years old."

Don't bother if you are planning to take estrogen replacement after menopause. Estrogen will protect your bones from losing mass for as long as you take it. But before you decide *not* to go on hormone therapy, you must find out if you are at high risk for osteoporosis by having your bones measured.

For younger women who are not on the brink of menopause, there's no reason for bone-density tests except in special circumstances such as a history of anorexia, long-term steroid treatments, malabsorption, or thyroid or parathyroid problems, all of which can lead to thinning bones.

"How does estrogen prevent bone loss?"

Estrogen increases the absorption of calcium by the bones and encourages bone formation, although it is not certain why. One theory is that it lowers the production of parathormone, a hormone made by the parathyroid gland, that normally increases with age and removes calcium from bone tissue. Another theory is that estrogen keeps bone destruction and bone formation in balance by suppressing the effect of interleukin-6, a chemical in the immune system that stimulates the growth of bone cells called osteoclasts. The osteoclasts' job is to find and remove old bone cells, while other cells, osteoblasts, are responsible for building new bone. When estrogen levels drop, the balance between osteoclasts and osteoblasts is disturbed, leading to more loss than gain.

"If I had menopause very early, at 35, when my ovaries were removed, do I have to be especially concerned about developing osteoporosis?"

Yes. Accelerated bone loss starts at menopause, no matter what age you have it. Women who have early menopause spend more years without estrogen than women who have it later, so they are at special risk for developing a serious case of brittle bones much sooner. Without estrogen replacement, you will have seventeen years of estrogen deficiency and bone loss behind you when you reach 52, the average age of menopause. Whether menopause occurs naturally or by surgical intervention, it's the number of years past menopause, not a woman's chronological age, that affects the strength of her bones.

"Is this especially true for women who have had surgical menopause?"

Yes. The abrupt and complete loss of estrogen can have a more serious impact on the rate of bone loss than the more gradual decline that accompanies natural menopause.

"I am 53 and had menopause five years ago. I recently had a bone-density test because my mother had osteoporosis and I was thinking of going on estrogen. I was told that I already have significant bone loss in my spine although not in other areas. Why is that?"

There are two types of bone: trabecular, the spongelike honey-combed network of porous bone that's found primarily in the spinal column, giving it great elasticity and strength; and cortical, the dense compact bone found predominantly in the legs and arms. Hips contain both trabecular and cortical bone.

With a deficiency of estrogen, the loss of bone tissue starts first in trabecular or vertebral bone, especially in the years immediately after menopause. Cortical bone, less sensitive to estrogen loss, catches up perhaps ten years down the road.

Sometimes osteoporosis is caused, not by estrogen deficiency, but by illness or long-term use of such drugs as corticosteroids, thyroid hormone, antacids that contain aluminum, heparin, tetracycline, anticonvulsants, isoniazid, oral antidiabetic drugs, and drugs used to suppress estrogen levels. Then the bone loss is more likely to show up first in cortical bone such as the hip.

In your case, unless there are important reasons for you not to take estrogen therapy, we recommend that you start it immediately to put a halt to the damage and to continue it for the rest of your life.

GETTING YOUR BONES MEASURED

There are several sophisticated screening techniques that can tell you the current status of your bones. They are reliable and painless and usually take about thirty minutes to perform. They include single photon absorpriometry (SPA), most commonly used to assess the density of the wrist and forearm, and dual photo absorptiometry (DPA), for evaluating the hip and spine. A newer technique is dual energy X-ray absorptiometry (DEXA), similar to DPA but more precise for measurements of both hip and spine. It provides an excellent technology for following the situation over time and monitoring the effectiveness of treatment.

Some physicians still rely on ordinary X-rays to diagnose osteoporosis. But while SPA or DEXA can detect bone loss of as little as 1 to 2 percent, standard X-rays don't pick up the damage until you have lost at least 25 to 30 percent of your bone. By then there's little you can do to improve the overall situation. An added benefit is that these new machines use extremely low doses of radiation. X-rays are useful, however, for ruling out other causes of back pain and to detect vertebral fractures in women with significant height loss but no other obvious symptoms.

Sometimes C/T scans (computerized tomography) with special attachments can provide excellent bone-density measurements, but because they require at least 9 rads of radiation (three times the amount for a standard chest X-ray and eighteen times the radiation needed for mammography) just to scan the spine, they are rarely used except in special cases.

A simpler test that can provide a clue to the presence of osteoporosis is the analysis of a twenty-four-hour urine sample for the ratio between calcium and an excreted substance called hydroxyproline. The results are an indication of whether calcium is being properly absorbed.

And, of course, a significant loss of height is an obvious indication of osteoporosis. If you are more than an inch and a half shorter than the height you started out as an adult, it has to be the result of spinal compression fractures caused by osteoporosis.

By the way, your measurements should always be made at the same time of day. All of us lose height—maybe three-quarters of an inch—during the day, probably from the loss of fluid in the spinal discs and the effect of gravity from a day in an erect position. After a night stretched out in bed, we are taller again in the morning.

THE OSTEOPOROSIS GENE: HAVE YOU GOT IT?

Heredity has long been known to play an important role in determining who gets osteoporosis, and an Australian research team has now linked a single gene to this disorder. If the studies prove valid, this discovery may lead to blood tests and other strategies in childhood that can help prevent brittle bones later.

The researchers say the normal gene's job is to produce a receptor protein in the body that helps vitamin D transport calcium into bone cells, making them strong and dense. If children grow up with a variation of the gene that prevents a proper hookup between the receptors and the hormone, they reach adulthood with bones that are significantly less dense than they should be and much more likely to fracture later.

If tests are developed to identify children with this genetic susceptibility to osteoporosis, preventive strategies could then be used. They include plenty of weight-bearing exercise and a diet rich in calcium and vitamin D.

PREVENTING OSTEOPOROSIS

There's no cure for osteoporosis, so your best defense is to build strong bones, starting *right now*, whatever your age. That means, first of all, that you consume enough calcium. If you are a typical American woman, it is most unlikely that you get a sufficient amount every day, especially if you are watching your weight. It's impossible to get that much calcium from food when you eat very few calories or avoid dairy products, especially as you get older and your absorption is not as efficient as it once was.

In contrast to other mineral nutrients such as sodium, potassium, and phosphate, calcium is not stored efficiently by the body for use during hard times. It plays a vital role in many day-to-day functions unrelated to bones, and it is lost every day through sweat, urine, feces, and shedding of skin cells. If you don't routinely consume and absorb enough calcium, it is stolen away from the bones and teeth to maintain a relatively constant supply in the bloodstream.

Check with your doctor if you take prescription or over-the-counter medications regularly, because some can have bone loss as a major side effect. These include some sedatives, antibiotics, steroids, thyroid hormone, cardiovascular therapies, Methotrexate, anticonvulsants, aluminum-containing antacids, and oral antidiabetic drugs.

Keep in mind that taking enough calcium is like putting money in the bank. By building your bones to their optimum strength as early as possible, you'll have something to fall back on when times get tough after menopause.

GOOD FOOD SOURCES OF CALCIUM

If you love milk—skim, low-fat, or whole—your problems are solved. If you don't, your next best bet is milk products such as low-fat cheese or yogurt—lots of them. Remember that not all dairy products are good calcium sources. Butter, cream cheese, and cream are high in fat and low in calcium.

Eat sardines or other soft-boned fish such as canned salmon, but be sure to include the bones. Tofu made with a calcium coagulant and other soybean products are other options. So is calcium-fortified orange juice, which usually provides 300 mg of calcium in an 8-ounce serving. (Skip the calcium-fortified "juice drinks," which contain minimal calcium and a lot of sugar.) Other fairly good calcium sources are dark green leafy vegetables such as collards, kale, and turnip greens. Even broccoli and lima beans contain significant amounts of calcium.

Spinach is a poor source because its high oxalic-acid content makes much of its calcium insoluble. Other leafy green vegetables that give you calcium but also the oxalic acid that interferes with its absorption are Swiss chard, sorrel, parsley, and beet greens. More foods high in oxalic acid include chocolate, rhubarb, peanuts, tea, and beans.

Some cereals are fortified with calcium. However, according to the Calcium Information Center, the fiber in cereal interferes with the absorption of calcium and therefore these products do not offer much benefit.

SCHEDULE FOR HEALTHY BONES

- *Birth to age 35:* This is when you have the opportunity to build your bones to their peak density and strength through a calcium-rich diet plus exercise.
- *Age 35 to 50 (or menopause):* Now the goal is to maintain the bone mass you've got. Be sure to take at least 1,000 mg of calcium a day, get weight-bearing exercise, limit alcohol to one or two drinks a day, stop smoking, stay away from drastic diets, and don't drink too much coffee.
- *Age 50 (or menopause) and over:* During the first few years after menopause, your bone density plummets and, to compound the problem, your calcium absorption becomes less efficient. Take at least 1,500 mg of calcium a day, continue to exercise, practice "clean living," and think seriously about starting hormone replacement therapy.

How Much Calcium Do You Need?

- Current opinion is that all women should consume 1,000 to 1,500 milligrams of calcium a day—the equivalent of three to five 8-ounce glasses of milk.
- Premenopausal women need at least 1,000 milligrams a day.
- Postmenopausal women require a minimum of 1,500 milligrams if they *don't* take estrogen, 1,000 milligrams a day if they *do.*

Most women don't eat anywhere near enough calcium-rich foods; in fact, studies have found that the majority of women at middle age and beyond take in no more than about 500 milligrams a day, with a third consuming less than 400 milligrams daily. If your dietary consumption is under the desirable limit for calcium intake, the intelligent thing to do is to take supplements.

Strong evidence of the value of calcium, especially after menopause, arrived in a recent two-year study conducted in New Zealand, which found that postmenopausal women who added 1,000 milligrams of calcium a day to what they were already getting in their food reduced their bone loss by 43 percent over women who took placebos. An additional benefit is that a calcium-fortified diet has been found to improve your cholesterol profile.

Lactose and vitamin D in milk and dairy products enhance the absorption of calcium, while fat decreases absorption and sodium increases its excretion, which means that less is retained by the bones. These are good reasons, aside from others, to limit your fat and salt intake.

Because magnesium is thought to play a role in the transport of calcium in and out of the body's cells, you should be sure you get enough of this mineral along with your calcium. A new study at Tel Aviv University's Sackler School of Medicine showed that bone loss can be prevented or even slightly reversed by magnesium supplements of 250 to 750 milligrams a day added to calcium supplements.

Calcium absorption requires adequate amounts, not only of vitamin D, but of A and C as well. So eating a balanced diet with a variety of foods and taking supplements where needed is your best protection (see table on page 78).

"I am lactose-intolerant, so I can't drink milk or eat milk products. How do I get enough calcium in my diet?"

You can't possibly get an adequate amount in your diet so you must take supplements. However, you might try some of these ways of getting around your lactose intolerance: take a lactase enzyme that may help you digest dairy foods; drink only a small amount of low-fat or skim milk at a time but adding up to several glasses a day; try lactose-reduced milk; try yogurt that contains active acidophilus cultures.

"I have to watch my weight all the time. I like milk but it is fattening. Do low-fat and skim milk contain as much calcium as whole milk?"

Yes, they and the dairy products made from them have as much calcium as whole-milk products. In fact, their concentration of calcium is even a little higher. We suggest you choose skim milk over low-fat because, once you get accustomed to it, it tastes just as good and we all should be consuming much less fat than we do.

"Is calcium-fortified orange juice a good way to get your calcium if you don't like to take pills?"

Certainly, if you can drink enough of it. A cup of calcium-rich orange juice usually contains about 300 milligrams of calcium.

Major Food Sources of Calcium

FOOD	SERVING SIZE	CALCIUM (MG)
Milk		
Evaporated, canned, unsweetened	½ cup	318
Low-fat (1%)	1 cup	298
Powdered, nonfat	¼ cup	384
Skim	1 cup	296
Whole	1 cup	288

FOOD	SERVING SIZE	CALCIUM (MG)
Yogurt		
Skim	1 cup	452
Low-fat (1%)	1 cup	415
Whole	1 cup	274
Cheese		
Hard (average)	1 ounce	212
Soft (average)	1 ounce	130
American, processed	1 ounce	196
Brie	1 ounce	52
Cheddar	1 ounce	214
Cottage, uncreamed	½ cup	88
Cottage, creamed	½ cup	109
Cream	2 tablespoons	23
Edam	1 ounce	225
Gruyère	1 ounce	308
Mozzarella	1 ounce	145
Provolone	1 ounce	212
Ricotta	½ cup	257
Swiss	1 ounce	260
Cheese spread, processed	1 ounce	159
Fish		
Salmon, canned, with bones	3 ounces	160
Sardines, canned, with bones	8 medium	354
Shrimp, canned	3½ ounces	115
Smelt, canned	4–5, medium	358
Meat Substitutes		
Tofu, soybean curd	4 ounces	152
Soybeans, cooked	½ cup	60
Vegetables		
Bok choy	½ cup	195

FOOD	SERVING SIZE	CALCIUM (MG)
Broccoli	½ cup	50
Collards	½ cup	179
Dandelion greens	½ cup	140
Kale	½ cup	103
Lima beans	½ cup	81
Mustard greens	½ cup	138
Rutabaga	½ cup	50
Fruits		
Blackberries	1 cup	46
Figs, dried	5 medium	126
Kumquats	5–6 medium	63
Orange	1 medium	58
Orange juice, calcium-fortified	6 ounces	220
Raisins, dried, seedless	½ cup	48
Nuts		
Almonds, shelled	½ cup	168
Brazil nuts, shelled	½ cup	130
Soybean nuts	½ cup	136
Sesame seeds	¼ cup	270
Desserts		
Custard	½ cup	140
Frozen yogurt	½ cup	100
Ice cream, plain	½ cup	98
Ice milk	½ cup	122
Pudding	½ cup	131
Tapioca pudding	½ cup	150

*Source: The Calcium Information Center, Barbara Levine, R.D., Ph.D., Director.

Don't Overdose on Vitamin D

Vitamin D and calcium work together as a team, but most people get plenty of vitamin D from sunlight and diet, especially from milk, which is usually fortified with it. Anywhere from 250 to 500 units a day is all you need; in fact, taking much more than that can be toxic. Many calcium supplements include this vitamin, so check the bottle to see if yours does before you decide to take more.

For most women, the only time to rely on vitamin D supplements (400 IU in a daily multivitamin tablet is plenty) is in the late winter in northern latitudes, when you are not likely to be exposed to much sunshine. Or, of course, if you are housebound or a workaholic who never gets out in the sun.

Some researchers also suggest that you take vitamin D supplements any time of the year after the age of about 65 or 70, especially if you don't take HRT, because aging reduces the capacity of the skin to use sunlight to produce the vitamin. They suggest 800 IU a day, although amounts larger than that may be toxic.

"I don't like taking drugs of any kind, including hormones, but I am worried about osteoporosis. Isn't it enough to take calcium supplements and get lots of exercise?"

No. Don't fool yourself into thinking that, if you stuff yourself with calcium and exercise for hours every week, you can prevent your bones from becoming more fragile. If you are a woman with an estrogen deficit, your bones cannot absorb and retain sufficient calcium to keep them at full strength. Depending on the skeleton you start out with, you can end up with brittle bones—the cause of all the humped backs and most of the broken hips you see among older women.

Don't get us wrong—you need plenty of calcium and weight-bearing exercise even if you begin with a sturdy frame and so can afford to lose some of it. You need it even more if your bones are fragile. But if you are a high-risk candidate for osteoporosis, *you absolutely cannot save your bones with calcium and/or exercise alone.* You need estrogen replacement. That's why HRT is almost universally recommended for all postmenopausal women who can use it safely.

"But I am taking the suggested quantity of calcium, 1,500 milligrams a day. That should be enough to keep anybody's bones strong."

Calcium is not a substitute for estrogen. Bone loss is so rapid in the years just after menopause, especially for some women, that taking lots of calcium can help slow down the rate of bone loss but it won't stop it. Even taking huge doses won't change your ultimate bone density, although it may retard the loss initially.

On the other hand, even with estrogen's help, you have to have enough of this mineral available for absorption by the bones. Going on hormone replacement at menopause, staying on it for life, *and* taking in adequate calcium through food and/or supplements give you the best chance of having strong bones when you are 90.

"How much calcium should I take in supplements and what kind is best?"

You should take whatever amount makes up for the shortage in your diet. For practical purposes, let's assume you get about 500 milligrams a day from your food. That means taking at least another 500 milligrams in supplements if you are premenopausal or you have had menopause and have started hormone therapy. If you don't drink milk or eat a lot of dairy products, you will require more. And, if you are postmenopausal and don't take estrogen, you need at least 1,500 milligrams every day. Up to 2,000 milligrams a day are considered safe.

There is a bewildering array of calcium supplements on the market. The major criteria for choosing one are the amount of *available elemental calcium* per pill, dissolvability, and cost. So read the labels and make sure you are getting at least 200 (and preferably more) milligrams of available elemental calcium per tablet. With less concentrated sources, you will have to take more pills a day to end up with sufficient calcium.

Also, make sure the pills dissolve readily (see below) and check out the cost per day, which depends on how many tablets per day you require to meet your quota.

"I'm afraid to take much calcium because it's supposed to cause kidney stones. What can I do instead?"

For a long time it was thought that too much dietary calcium caused kidney stones because most stones are composed of calcium compounds. However, a recent study suggests just the opposite: calcium may help *prevent* kidney stones, at least among men (women were not included in the study). So take your calcium and don't worry about kidney stones.

Test Your Tablets

To be sure your calcium supplements are good quality, meaning that the calcium is bioavailable, easily dissolved, and absorbed by your body, test the tablets this way:

Place a tablet in a saucer and cover it with distilled white vinegar. Stir every few minutes. It should disintegrate or break up within twenty to thirty minutes. If the tablet is still in one piece after half an hour, try another brand.

Here are some don'ts about taking calcium supplements:

- Don't take a higher dose than recommended, unless you are under the supervision of a doctor. It causes constipation in some people, and excessive amounts may interfere with the body's ability to absorb iron and zinc. Also, consult your physician about possible interactions with prescription or over-the-counter medications.
- Avoid taking calcium with high-fiber meals or with bulk-forming laxatives because the fiber reduces absorption.
- Don't take calcium with iron pills or multivitamins containing high iron because calcium interferes with iron absorption.
- Drink plenty of fluids—six to eight glasses a day.

CHOICES IN CALCIUM SUPPLEMENTS

Calcium carbonate, the most commonly used supplement, is easily absorbed, has the highest percentage of elemental calcium per tablet (40 percent), and is the least expensive. Its disadvantage is that it sometimes causes uncomfortable side effects such as bloating, gas, and constipation. Also, because it has a buffering effect on the stomach, it may reduce the bioavailability of iron.

Tricalcium phosphate provides about the same available elemental calcium per tablet, but on the other hand, it tends not to have the same gas-producing effect.

Calcium citrate, usually available today in microcrystalline form, is the most soluble and absorbable form of calcium, although it contains about half as much bioavailable calcium per tablet as calcium carbonate and tricalcium phosphate, and therefore costs more for the same dose. It is the kind usually found in calcium-fortified orange juice. Calcium citrate will dissolve in less stomach acid than other calcium compounds, so it may be a better choice for people with achlorhydria, or decreased stomach acid—a common condition in older people.

Calcium lactate and *calcium gluconate*, with only about a quarter of the elemental calcium per tablet of that supplied by calcium carbonate, are also more expensive because they require more tablets per dose. However, they are usually tolerated well.

Bonemeal or *dolomite*, natural sources of calcium, are not advised because they may be contaminated with significant amounts of lead or other toxic metals.

Oyster shell calcium is natural, which appeals to many women, and is a good source of calcium carbonate. However, there's no need to pay more for it—the synthetic form is chemically identical and just as effective.

Chelated calcium is also more expensive and is not absorbed better than other supplements.

Antacids such as Tums, Tums E-X, and Rolaids Calcium Rich are good sources, although you will require several tablets a day to meet your requirements, which raises the cost. And they come in flavors. Be sure to avoid antacids that contain aluminum because these have the opposite effect on calcium absorption than you are looking for. Antacids that contain magnesium, such as Maalox, may be good to take in combination with calcium because they help prevent constipation.

"When's the best time to take the calcium supplements?"

To boost absorption, always take calcium supplements with food, after a meal or even a small snack, when the stomach's production of hydrochloric acid is at its peak. Don't take it late at night on an empty stomach because it could be irritating. If you have too little stomach acid, like many older people, take calcium lactate or calcium citrate. Or take it with citrus juice, which increases absorption because the acidity of the juice helps dissolve the tablets.

Take no more than 600 milligrams of elemental calcium at any one time, or over 2,000 milligrams in one day, to diminish the possibilities of gastric reactions. Besides, you can absorb only that much at a time and the rest will be excreted. It's best to space the supplements in several doses throughout the day with your food.

"I am very confused about how much actual calcium I'm getting in my calcium supplements. How do I figure it out?"

All supplements are a compound of calcium with other elements. You're interested in the amount of elemental calcium listed on the label because that's the amount the supplement can deliver. In general, if a product label states that each tablet contains 500 milligrams of calcium, that means it provides 500 milligrams of elemental calcium. But if it states only that it contains 500 milligrams of calcium carbonate, for example, then you must know what percentage of that is elemental calcium. In this case, each tablet contains 200 milligrams of elemental calcium because there is 40 percent calcium in calcium carbonate.

"I eat lots of whole grains and legumes but I have read that the phytic acid in them interferes with the absorption of calcium. Is that true?"

Yes. Both phytates and oxalates (in spinach and other leafy greens) block absorption of calcium in those foods. Not only that, but a high-fiber diet, currently held in high esteem, can also result in excessive calcium excretion, meaning that your bones may not absorb enough of this important nutrient. If you are essentially a vegetarian, that's great, but for the sake of your bones, be sure to eat large amounts of dairy foods and take sufficient supplements.

"What about dieting? I've heard this is bad for bones, too."

Women on any diet that reduces their caloric intake sharply, even when they exercise and consume adequate amounts of calcium, tend to lose bone mass. High-protein diets (also called high-ash diets), so popular a couple of decades ago, are notorious for causing loss of bone tissue. In fact, we are now seeing amazing numbers of women who went on and off those diets for years at a time, and thereby added another major risk factor for osteoporosis because they lost bone along with the weight. Too much protein causes acidosis—a higher-than-normal concentration of acid in the blood—which promotes calcium depletion from the bones.

Dieting or not, the average woman in the United States eats two to three times as much protein as she needs. If you are in this category, it may help your skeleton if you started eating a more balanced diet.

"I have always been very overweight, even obese at times. Is it true that I'm not as likely to have osteoporosis later on?"

Yes, it's true, although this is the only good thing we can think of to say about obesity. Very overweight women tend to be at a lower risk for brittle bones, probably because some estrogen continues to be converted from adrenal hormones in the adipose (fat) tissue. In most cases, the greater the body fat, the greater the estrogen production even after menopause. Also, excess weight increases the mechanical load on the bones, helping to strengthen them.

"What drugs and medications affect the absorption or retention of calcium?"

Cholestyramine, tetracycline antibiotics, heparin, corticosteroids, many furosemide diuretics, anticonvulsant drugs, muscle relaxants, sedatives, some oral antidiabetic agents, and excessive levels of thyroid hormone affect absorption or retention of calcium. Also, some of the bulk-producing therapeutic fiber preparations do the same.

"Can osteoporosis affect my teeth?"

Definitely. It can cause a loss of bone in the jaw, shrinking the sockets that hold your teeth firmly in place.

"I don't understand how smoking can possibly be a risk factor for osteoporosis. How does it affect your bones?"

Smoking is probably the worst thing you can do for every part of your body, including your skeleton, where it robs the bones of their mineral density. It is bad for bones because it interferes with the body's production of estrogen. And if you're on estrogen therapy after menopause, it can cancel out the hormone's protection against fractures.

Not only that, but smoking can cause an earlier menopause, giving you more years of estrogen deficiency and therefore more opportunity to develop osteoporosis as you get older. Bone loss is about twice as rapid among thin postmenopausal women who are heavy cigarette smokers than among thin postmenopausal women who don't smoke.

Researchers at the University of Melbourne in Australia, who recently studied the connection between smoking and osteoporosis, calculated that if a woman smoked a pack of cigarettes a day throughout adulthood, her bones would be 5 to 10 percent less dense than they otherwise would have been at menopause.

"And coffee too? Do I have to give up all my bad habits to defend my bones?"

A lifetime of coffee drinking may decrease your bone density, although a daily glass of milk can offset that loss, according to recent research at the University of California, San Diego. The research shows that drinking as little as two cups of caffeinated coffee a day results in a significant decline in bone density as you get older—unless you also drink milk—but the more coffee you drink, the less milk you are likely to consume. Previous research showed that caffeine increases urinary excretion of calcium.

So safe guidelines probably are to drink no more than two cups of coffee, three cups of tea, or four diet sodas in one day. *And* to increase your consumption of milk. The scientists found that women who consumed two or more cups of coffee daily and at least one glass of milk a day for about forty years had bone density 6.5 percent higher than women who drank the coffee and didn't drink milk.

"What about decaffeinated coffee?"

We don't know because the study did not include women who drank only decaffeinated coffee.

"And soft drinks?"

Some research points to diet soda as another potential villain because the phosphorus they contain is thought to steal calcium away from bones and teeth. But soft drinks probably don't contain enough phosphorus to do damage.

"I enjoy a cocktail before dinner, but I've heard that alcohol can promote osteoporosis. What are the facts? Do I have to give up alcohol?"

One or two drinks a day aren't going to affect your bones; in fact, they may even be good for your heart (although possibly bad for your breast-cancer risk). But heavy drinkers lose bone at a faster rate than moderate drinkers or teetotalers, probably because alcohol inhibits calcium retention. Besides, people who seriously overindulge usually have poor eating habits.

EXERCISE AND YOUR BONES

Exercise plays a definite role in maximizing peak bone mass in your younger days and in reducing its loss as you get older. Bones are like muscles—if you use them, they get stronger and thicker, especially when you are young. Exercise not only builds bone but also increases muscle mass, which can protect against fractures by absorbing the shock of a fall. Moreover, it improves your coordination, balance, and strength, making you less likely to fall down and break something.

ANTIGRAVITATIONAL IS WHAT YOU NEED

Almost any kind of exercise makes you more fit, strengthens your heart and lungs, gives you flexibility and endurance, tones up your muscles, and makes you feel more mentally alert. But to maintain healthy bones, you must do a certain *kind* of physical activity. This means weight-bearing antigravitational exercise such as walking, jogging, aerobics, biking, stair climbing, racquet sports, dancing, and any form of running and jumping; also activities like weight lifting that involve high loads and high stresses. The exercise must stress the spine and the long bones of the body and add the force of gravity.

The good news is that just plain brisk walking is as effective for this purpose as any other antigravitational exercise. Many women consider a slow stroll around the shopping mall to be sufficient. It isn't. It can't hurt, and any exercise is better than none, especially for women who have never moved very much before. But to do much good for your bones or the rest of you, you must walk fast enough to cover three miles in less than an hour, and you must do it often.

Although your bone-building days were over when you reached 30 or 35, it's important now to protect the bone you've got. Exercise helps, especially when it is used in combination with increased calcium intake and, after menopause, with hormone replacement therapy. One study concluded that, along with 1,000 milligrams of calcium added to their daily diets, one group of postmenopausal women controlled bone loss with a one-hour low-impact aerobics class and two brisk thirty-minute walks a week.

Although exercise is only part of the formula for keeping your bones in good condition for the rest of your life, it is an important element. So make it a routine part of your life to include moderately vigorous weight-bearing activities for at least a half hour four times a week.

"Is the beneficial effect of exercise on bones lost if you stop doing it?"

Yes. In fact, it is lost very quickly when you diminish the intensity and frequency of your physical activity and take up a sedentary lifestyle.

"Is it wise to exercise after a bone-density test has shown that you've got osteoporosis? I am feeling very fragile and am afraid to do very much."

It's even more important now to get enough exercise, especially the weight-bearing kind such as brisk walking, because it gives you muscle strength and strengthens your skeleton. Of course, it makes sense to avoid potentially jarring exercise, like skiing, if your osteoporosis is advanced. It's important, too, to consume plenty of calcium and, if it is not contraindicated in your case, to start taking estrogen supplements immediately.

"How do I know if I am estrogen-deficient?"

Every woman is deficient in estrogen after menopause. By definition, this is the time when hormone production is drastically diminished, and without estrogen's help, your bones cannot possibly retain all of their solidity and strength. That's one major reason why hormone replacement therapy is almost universally recommended for most postmenopausal women with fragile bone structures.

As long as your ovaries continue to produce estrogen—the major female hormone—you will maintain a fairly good balance between bone loss and bone replacement. After menopause, however, you won't. You will start losing bone mass at an accelerated pace, especially in the first seven to ten years. What this means, especially if you are a high-risk candidate for osteoporosis, is that you need estrogen replacement starting *immediately* after menopause. The minimum dosage for prevention of osteoporosis is usually .625 milligram of conjugated estrogen a day or the equivalent, but some need more. On the other hand, petite women may get adequate blood levels of estrogen with even smaller doses. That's why HRT must be individualized.

Hormone replacement is the single most effective way to prevent osteoporosis, and the National Institutes of Health is now recommending that all women consider it after menopause. It is, in fact, the *only* way to prevent bone loss. It can actually increase your bone mass in the first three years, and then stop you from losing any more.

"How long do I have to stay on HRT to preserve my bones?"

To prevent osteoporosis permanently, estrogen replacement must be a long-term commitment. It works only as long as you take it. If you take it for several years and then quit, the bone loss will begin again and will be especially rapid for a few years after you stop, just as it would have immediately after menopause if you had never taken it. However, for whatever time you have been on HRT, you have maintained your bone density and now your bones are that much sturdier than they would otherwise have been. To maintain your bones all of your life, however, you must take HRT all of your life.

"I read in the newspaper that women aren't any better off at age 75 whether or not they took HRT earlier for a few years. Their bones show no difference in density, so why bother?"

If you take HRT for ten years starting at age 50 and then stop, your bones will be stronger longer than they will be for women who have never taken estrogen. But they will gradually lose their density after you quit taking estrogen; so, by the time you are 75 or 80, you will probably have lost that extra protection. To have the strongest possible bones all of your life, you must start taking estrogen at the time of menopause and never stop.

"Is it ever too late to start?"

No matter when you start taking estrogen regularly, it will keep osteoporosis from advancing further. So even if you did not start at menopause, you will benefit by taking it later.

What You Must Remember

- HRT helps protect your bones only as long as you take it. When you stop the therapy, bone loss resumes.
- The sooner after menopause you start taking estrogen, the less bone you will lose.
- Even if you start taking estrogen later, you will have a better chance to benefit because it will stop further bone loss.

"Does progesterone, the hormone I'm supposed to take along with estrogen, counteract estrogen's effect on bones?"

No, just the opposite. Recent studies have found that taking progesterone actually increases the effect, producing even thicker and stronger bone tissue than estrogen alone.

Once More, No Smoking!

Smoking wipes out estrogen therapy's preventive effect on bone fractures, according to researchers at Brown University School of Medicine. Among 2,873 women studied, the risk for hip fracture was substantially greater in current smokers on hormones than in women on hormones who had never been addicted to cigarettes. The risk was higher, too, in women who had *ever* smoked. So, if you smoke cigarettes, don't bother to take HRT to forestall osteoporosis. You will have already cancelled out its protection.

What's more, smokers' bones heal more slowly because the smoke reduces oxygen flow to the tissues. A three-year study recently reported to the American Academy of Orthopedic Surgeons concludes that broken bones take about five months longer to mend for smokers than nonsmokers.

"I have been told I can't take estrogen therapy because of previous breast cancer and, besides, I am taking tamoxifen to block the estrogen I make. Isn't tamoxifen supposed to prevent osteoporosis too?"

Tamoxifen is actually a weak estrogen. It acts like an estrogen in some areas of the body—such as the bones and the heart—and as an estrogen blocker in other areas, such as the vagina and the brain. It does good things for the bones and, judging from the results of early studies, seems to be just as good for preventing osteoporosis as estrogen. You must be vigilant, however, about getting gynecological checkups regularly because tamoxifen seems to increase the risk of getting cancer of the uterus.

"Does the transdermal patch do as good a job in preventing osteoporosis as oral estrogen?"

Just as good. The most recent evidence shows that the results are the same whether the estrogen is delivered by pill or by patch, and the FDA has recently approved the patch "for use in the prevention of postmenopausal osteoporosis." Both maintain bone density, so it doesn't matter which you choose. Vaginal estrogen cream, however, although it is effective to some extent, should not be relied upon to preserve your bones.

"I am 37 and have been taking steroids for two years because of my arthritis. Now I've found out steroids cause osteoporosis. What should I do?"

Taking steroids for a few weeks here and there won't affect your bone tissue, but chronic use can cause dramatic bone loss. So can high doses of thyroid hormone. A recent study on a group of patients taking prednisone found that the longer the steroids were used and the higher the dosage, the greater the loss of bone. So have your bone density measured periodically to determine your status. Take extra calcium and vitamin D now, and when you have menopause, be sure your doctor prescribes replacement therapy immediately.

ALTERNATIVE THERAPIES FOR OSTEOPOROSIS

For women who can't take estrogen because they have had breast cancer but are already suffering from symptomatic osteoporosis, there are a few alternatives that may help them fend off more bone loss. All of them have their problems and none is as effective as estrogen.

SALMON CALCITONIN

A synthetic hormone, salmon calcitonin is the only drug other than estrogen that has been approved by the FDA for the treatment of osteoporosis. It is used exclusively for its effects on bone tissue and is now the primary alternative treatment for women who can't take estrogen or choose not to use it after menopause. Used in conjunction with adequate calcium and vitamin D intake, it maintains bone mass and, at the same time, has a pain-relieving effect.

About a third of the women who take calcitonin have problems tolerating its side effects (nausea, diarrhea, metallic taste, flushing, and sometimes a rash) as it is currently administered—by injection daily or at least three times a week. But a calcitonin nasal spray, already in use in many other countries and recently submitted for approval by the FDA, promises to eliminate the unpleasant side effects along with the needles. Meanwhile, try injecting the medication at bedtime or ask your doctor if you might reduce the dose temporarily to see if that will help.

ETIDRONATE

Combined with calcium, etidronate (Didronel) can increase bone mass and cut the incidence of spinal fractures by half for women who already suffer from significant osteoporosis. Etidronate appears to work on the spine (it does not have the same effect on cortical bone such as the hip) by coating bone cells and preventing loss of bone tissue. However, this drug has not yet been approved for this use by the FDA, and its long-term effects on the body are not yet determined. We do know that etidronate must be taken in a very careful start-

and-stop fashion or it will cause more harm than good. It must be taken for no longer than two weeks at a time, followed by ten to twelve weeks of heavy calcium loading.

SODIUM FLUORIDE

Once thought to be an answer for treating osteoporosis, sodium fluoride has been used for many years because it stimulates bone cells and increases bone density in the spine, probably by encouraging the retention of calcium. The hope was that it would therefore reduce spinal fractures. But a Mayo Clinic study, among others, found that while fluoride supplementation does increase bone tissue, the new bone tends to be structurally abnormal—more like a hard collagen substance—and is therefore more brittle than normal bone.

Besides, sodium fluoride has many unpleasant side effects, such as gastrointestinal symptoms, leg pain, anemia, and nausea. Its use remains controversial, although a slow-releasing form of sodium fluoride that has minimal side effects and produces stronger bone currently looks promising. In April 1994, researchers at the University of Texas Southwestern Medical Center at Dallas released interim findings of an ongoing experiment that seem to show that low doses of fluoride given in slow-release form along with a readily absorbed type of calcium can reduce spinal fractures in older women with osteoporosis by about half after about two and a half years. The treatment also increased bone mass slightly. The women were given two doses of fluoride and two of calcium daily for 12 months, followed by two months without the fluoride before beginning the regime again.

CALCITRIOL

Another experimental drug for osteoporotic women who can't take estrogen is calcitriol. A new study of over 400 women who had moderate osteoporosis compared the effects of calcitriol, a synthetic form of vitamin D, with calcium supplements taken for three years. The women on calcitriol had a threefold reduction in the rate of new spinal fractures as compared to women on calcium.

FOSAMAX

An investigational drug in a new family of compounds known as amino-biphosphonates, Fosamax (alendronate sodium) is not yet on the market, but a two-year clinical study has shown that it can increase bone density in the spine and hip of postmenopausal women with osteoporosis.

Chapter 5

YOUR HEART: KEEPING IT HEALTHY

THE HEALTHIER YOUR HEART AND ARTERIES ARE NOW, and the more you work at keeping them that way, the better they will serve you for the rest of your life. So plan ahead. A few practical precautions now can pay off enormously in the long term.

Most women seem to think that heart attacks are reserved for men, although the truth is that heart disease doesn't discriminate. It strikes women just as often as men. And although most women are much more afraid of breast cancer than a heart attack, they are five times more likely to die of a cardiovascular complication than of cancer. Heart disease is, in fact, the number one killer and a leading disabler of women.

Women do have one important advantage over men when it comes to the heart. They develop the first signs of coronary artery disease (CAD) about ten or fifteen years later in life than men and tend to be, on average, twenty years older when they experience a first heart attack. It is very rare for a woman to have a heart attack before the age of 50—in other words, before menopause—unless she has uncontrolled hypertension, diabetes, or congenital heart disease. But after-

99

wards, the risk steadily climbs each year, and by the age of 65, a woman's chances are the same as a man's at 55. At 72, the risks for men and women merge and become about equal.

But if a woman has an early menopause or has her ovaries removed before their time, she doesn't get the ten-year advantage over men. Whatever her age, she promptly moves into the higher risk group as soon as her ovaries stop producing estrogen.

YOUR FEMALE HORMONES PROTECT YOU

Nobody knows for sure why women don't get heart disease as early as men, but the protection almost certainly comes from estrogen, the major female hormone. After menopause, this protection quickly vanishes and, together with the changes that normally occur with age, allows the rate of stroke and heart attack to climb.

This premise is strengthened by the fact that women who take hormone replacement therapy after menopause tend to live significantly longer than those who don't. One major study by the National Institutes of Health found that the death rate for women on HRT was only a third as high as that for other women, with the most pronounced difference in life span among women whose ovaries had been removed before menopause. Another large study involving nearly 49,000 nurses concluded that women who take estrogen after menopause cut their risk of heart disease almost in half.

As for stroke, the number three cause of death for women, yet another group of researchers analyzed data from almost 1,910 postmenopausal women collected over an average of almost twelve years and concluded that "overall, postmenopausal hormone use resulted in a 31 percent reduction in the incidence of stroke and in a 63 percent reduction in death caused by stroke."

HOW ESTROGEN DOES THE JOB

Researchers speculate that at least part of estrogen's protective effect comes from its ability to raise the level of HDL that clears plaque and fatty streaks from the arteries, while also decreasing LDL (low-density lipoprotein) that encourages accumulation of plaque. *In fact, estrogen is believed to have a* more *profound effect in altering the HDL to LDL ratio than any cholesterol-lowering drug yet discovered.*

Some studies also suggest that estrogen may work directly to clear deposits from arterial walls, inhibit platelet aggregation, maintain the elasticity of the arteries, and increase arterial blood flow by dilating the small arteries. But however it works, there's overwhelming evidence that HRT significantly reduces a postmenopausal woman's risk of stroke and heart disease, especially if she already has coronary artery disease (CAD).

"I've heard that progesterone cancels out the beneficial effects of estrogen on the heart and arteries. Is this true?"

There has been plenty of evidence that estrogen helps offset the increased risk of heart disease that normally accompanies menopause, but also considerable concern that adding progesterone to protect against uterine cancer might cancel out that important effect. According to a couple of recent studies, however, the prospects are good that the combination therapy is just as beneficial for the heart as estrogen is on its own.

For example, a team led by University of Michigan researchers studied over 5,000 postmenopausal women. They found that the cholesterol levels of women taking both hormones were just as good as those who took estrogen alone, concluding that both regimens reduced the risk of CAD by about 40 percent.

Other researchers, this time from the DeBakey Heart Center in Houston, reported in 1994 that taking estrogen and progesterone together reduces by 50 percent the level of a form of "bad cholesterol" called Lp(a), which increases the risk of blocked arteries. The combination produces the same increase in HDL and decrease in LDL cholesterol that estrogen alone does, probably because both hormones make the liver more efficient in removing the harmful cholesterol from the bloodstream.

A third study, published in late 1994 by Dr. Trudy Bush, an epidemiologist at Johns Hopkins School of Medicine, and Dr. Elizabeth Barrett-Connor, at the University of California in San Diego, provides further confirmation that progesterone combined with estrogen is just as good for the heart as estrogen alone. And adds two other reassuring findings: that combination therapy protected women against uterine cancer and did not increase the risk of breast cancer.

Consider This

Your chances of dying of AIDS are 1 in a million. Your chances of dying in an automobile accident are 1 in 10,000 per year. Your chances of dying of cancer are 1 in 5. Your chances of dying of cardiovascular disease, however, are 1 in *2*.

SO WHAT'S A WOMAN TO DO?

If you haven't yet had menopause, begin protecting your heart now so that when your estrogen supply closes down you will be off to a good start. Even if you have no family history of heart disease, at least follow the four pillars of prevention: stop smoking, control hypertension, eat to lower cholesterol and obesity, and exercise.

If you have had menopause, the advice here becomes even more important because you have already lost the special protection that comes with being a menstruating woman who makes plenty of her own hormones.

Stop Smoking Smoking is the worst thing you can do to your heart. It constricts the arteries, increases clotting, and reduces the oxygen supply to the heart muscle. It also releases substances into the blood that damage artery walls, thicken them, and make them more prone to plaque deposits. As few as one to four cigarettes a day doubles your risk of heart disease and more than that increases it further. If you quit, no matter how long you have been a smoker, you will reduce your risk by half in only a year.

Quitting can reduce your heart attack risk 50 to 70 percent.

Watch Your Weight Overweight is bad for anybody's health, but women are much more likely to be obese than men. Women who are more than 30 percent above their ideal weight raise their risk of heart disease because obesity not only overstresses the heart but increases susceptibility to diabetes, high levels of "bad" LDL cholesterol, and elevated blood pressure—all risk factors in themselves. However, it's important to lose weight sensibly; in other words, take it off gradually and then keep it off.

Change Your Sedentary Habits High levels of physical fitness are associated with a lower risk of heart disease in both women and men. According to the findings of a large study at the Institute for Aerobics Research in Dallas, sedentary women were nine times more likely to die from cardiovascular disease than were those who were most fit. Elsewhere, researchers found that regular exercisers had arteries that were about a third less rigid than their more sedentary counterparts. And very recent research finds that regular exercise strongly protects you against a heart attack set off by a sudden burst of physical activity, such as running for the bus or shoveling snow.

Any amount or variety of exercise is better than none at all, especially if you don't move very much now. A brisk half-hour walk, a bike ride, or some gardening can have a real impact. But, of course, it's much better to get regular exercise that raises your heart rate to at least 50 percent of its maximum capacity (see Chapter 19).

What's the Exercise Payoff?

The payoff is a longer, healthier life. Among the cardiovascular benefits of regular exercise are a diminished tendency of the blood to form clots, an improved cholesterol profile, more efficient use of oxygen by the muscles, a larger volume of blood pumped with each heartbeat, and, during periods of exertion, greater dilation of the arteries, lower heart rate, and lower blood pressure. Exercise also delays the rigidity that tends to afflict our arteries as we get older and heads off strokes.

Regulate Your Cholesterol Level   The total cholesterol numbers are not as important for women as are the ratio between LDLs, which encourage the deposit of arterial plaque, and HDLs, whose job is to carry that plaque away. Estrogen tends to keep HDLs elevated in women until after menopause, when HDL levels drop thereby increasing the risk of cardiovascular disease. As for triglycerides (fats in the blood that are transported with the cholesterol), their role is still controversial. A high level is thought to raise the risk of cardiovascular disorders, especially when it accompanies diabetes.

Watch Out for Diabetes   Diabetes—which affects about twice as many women as men after age 45 and has a more devastating effect on women—is a major contributor to CAD because high blood sugar increases triglyceride levels and leads to hardening of the arteries. Women who develop diabetes lose their natural ten- or fifteen-year grace period and end up with an even higher chance of developing heart disease at the same age as men and, besides, are more likely to die from it. A diabetic woman's chances of having a heart attack is two to three times that of a nondiabetic.

The usual onset of the most common form of diabetes is over the age of 40 to 45. You can lower your risk of getting diabetes by keeping your weight down and exercising regularly. If you are already diabetic, it is absolutely essential to keep your glucose levels under very tight control.

Control Your Blood Pressure   Chronically elevated blood pressure raises the chances of coronary disease and heart attacks and is the single biggest risk factor for strokes, although women seem to tolerate hypertension better than men. Fewer women die from complications compared to men and fewer women also go on to develop a more serious, untreatable kind of hypertension. However, the longer you live with hypertension, the worse the condition of your arteries is likely to become. Have your doctor check your blood pressure regularly; if it is elevated, work on lowering it with lifestyle changes and, if necessary, drugs. Half of all hypertensive women are obese, and when overweight hypertensive women reduce their weight, their blood pressure goes down.

By the way, the most frequently found reversible cause of hypertension is overconsumption of alcohol. If you are a drinker who has been recently diagnosed as having high blood pressure, cut out the alcohol and get tested again.

Eat Preventively   Reduce your total fat intake to less than 30 percent of your diet if you have no family history of heart disease. Reduce it more drastically—to 20 or 25 percent, or less if you can manage it, perhaps even switching to a vegetarian diet—if you have inherited heart problems or already have evidence of disease. Cut down especially severely on animal fats and limit any kind of saturated fat to no more than 10 percent of your total diet. Substitute monosaturated fats such as olive oil as much as possible. Increase your consumption of fruits, vegetables, grains—especially those containing antioxidant vitamins.

Consume Antioxidants   There is more and more evidence that a simple and safe preventive against heart attacks and artery damage is a diet that includes large amounts of the antioxidant vitamins C, E, and beta-carotene. Antioxidants are substances that block the oxidation of harmful LDL cholesterol, thereby inhibiting the accumulation of plaque in the arteries. Although all the facts are not yet in, it seems eminent good sense to concentrate on foods that contain these vitamins and, in addition, to take supplements. For details, see page 109.

Consume Folic Acid   A series of recent studies suggest that this B vitamin (also called folacin or folate) may help ward off heart attacks, strokes, and even cancer. Few of us eat enough of it in our daily diets—it is found in liver, dark green leafy vegetables, some nuts, seeds, and grains, legumes, fortified cereals, some fruits and vegetables—to get the 400 micrograms a day that is currently recommended. So we suggest getting your allotted amount in a supplement.

Take HRT   One big advantage women have over men is that they can take hormone replacement therapy when their own hormone production diminishes and their susceptibility to heart disease rises. In postmenopausal women at high risk for CAD, estrogen therapy cuts the risk by as much as half.

Know Your Family History If close relatives have CAD or have had a heart attack, especially before the age of 50, be sure to have routine screenings at regular intervals.

One in nine women aged 45 to 65 has some form of heart disease or stroke. This ratio soars to one in three at age 65 and beyond, according to the American Heart Association.

FAST FACTS ABOUT THE FEMALE HEART

- It may take longer for women to start getting heart disease, but when they do, it is a far more serious event than it is for men. According to the American Heart Association, when a woman has a heart attack she is twice as likely as a man to die within the first sixty days. Moreover, 39 percent of women who suffer heart attacks die within a year (vs. 31 percent of men). After that, a woman is twice as likely to have a second heart attack as a man.
- About 500,000 American women die of cardiovascular disease every year.
- Black women are one and a half times more likely than white women to have fatal heart attacks. They also have a higher prevalence of hypertension and its malevolent effects.
- More than half of all women eventually develop some form of heart disease. One out of every two women dies from it.
- About 30 percent of women under 55, and 50 percent over 55, have high cholesterol levels, says the American Medical Association's Women's Health Campaign. About half of women over 55 have high blood

pressure; 30 percent of white women and 50 percent of black women are classified as obese; and 60 percent of women lead sedentary lifestyles, exercising less than twenty minutes three times a week.

• Female heart patients are generally much sicker than men by the time they get treatment, and are often treated less aggressively. They are much less likely to be treated with the most up-to-date care and with procedures such as cardiac catheterization (a diagnostic procedure that determines the severity of artery blockage), angiograms, balloon angioplasty, or coronary bypass.

Is this the result of discrimination? Often, but not always. Women are typically ten to fifteen years older than men when they develop heart disease and doctors are often reluctant to recommend invasive tests and procedures for frail elderly patients. Besides, about 10 percent of women with coronary symptoms turn out to have normal major coronary arteries that are free of atherosclerosis and suffer instead from smaller vessel spasm. Also, women tend to have such small coronary vessels that they may not be ideal candidates for bypass surgery or angioplasty. And last, many diagnostic tests have limited usefulness in women. Stress tests, for example, are associated with close to 45 percent false-positive results in women.

• Until recently, women have been almost completely excluded from studies of CAD. In addition, many researchers have excluded people over 65, the age when women are most likely to suffer from heart disease.

• Even at the same age, women with heart disease tend to receive less care than men, possibly because physicians, expecting to find less heart disease among them, may attribute their symptoms to other causes.

• The symptoms of a heart attack are often less pronounced in women than in men, and painless heart attacks among them occur more frequently. This is especially true for diabetic women whose neuropathy (nerve damage) may make them less sensitive to cardiac pain.

• Women who have early menopause—and who do not take hormone replacement therapy—tend to have an earlier and higher incidence of heart disease.

"How important is family history as a risk factor for heart disease?"

Very important. If, for example, one of your parents had a heart attack, your risk is doubled. A family history of hypertension or early heart disease—especially on your maternal side and especially before the age of 50—also increases your risk. It becomes especially vital for you to make sure you are doing your best to eliminate preventable risk factors.

"Shouldn't everyone go on a salt-free diet to prevent high blood pressure and heart disease?"

Not at all. Many people today needlessly limit their salt intake, thinking salt is dangerous for them. But the vast majority of people tolerate salt very well and don't have to worry about it.

Only about 20 percent of the population has to be concerned about keeping salt consumption low because of hypertension, congestive heart failure, a rare adrenal hormone disease, or some kinds of kidney disease.

"My friend takes a lot of vitamins every day as a protection, she says, against a heart attack. What are the facts?"

If those vitamins are antioxidants, your friend may be absolutely correct, according to rapidly accumulating scientific evidence. Several recent studies have shown that antioxidants—vitamin E, vitamin C, beta-carotene (a parent molecule of vitamin A), and other substances such as selenium—can protect against coronary disease by preventing cholesterol deposits from forming on artery walls. Vitamin E may prove to be the most effective, according to the newest research.

A recent study of women indicated that those who consumed large amounts of beta-carotene and vitamin E had substantially less heart disease than women who consumed less. Another study found that daily doses of at least 100 units of vitamin E for two years or more cut the risk of heart disease among women by 46 percent. Adding to the evidence, two other reports—from the Harvard School of Public Health and Brigham and Women's Hospital—linked daily supplements of 100 or more units of vitamin E with about a 40 percent reduction in major coronary events for both men and women.

Beta-carotene reduced the death rate from heart disease by 40 to 50 percent in a group of elderly people, and the more they consumed, the lower their risk. Tests with vitamin C have shown similar results.

Vitamin C appears to reduce death rates from heart disease among both men and women by as much as an average of 36 percent, according to the results of a study at the University of California, Los Angeles, of the diets of more than 11,000 American adults.

"I've read about a 1994 Finnish study that showed the anti-oxidant vitamins didn't help prevent cancer and heart disease and, in fact, may even be harmful. What do you say about that?"

We definitely lean in favor of taking the vitamins because of the weight of the considerable research that has found significant reductions in heart disease among those who took the supplements. The study you cite involved men over the age of 50 who were long-term smokers, people who probably already had artery and heart damage before the research began. We suggest taking the vitamins as a preventive measure, not as a cure. In the meantime, more studies of these supplements are underway in women as well as men, using lower doses taken over a longer time. Eventually, we will have definitive answers to the question of their effectiveness.

"How can these vitamins provide protection against heart disease?"

Scientists believe that free radicals—substances made by the body when it uses oxygen—not only cause harmful aging changes in cells and tissues but also are required for the oxidation of harmful low-density lipoprotein (LDL) cholesterol. Once the LDL is oxidized, it is more easily taken up in artery walls, thereby narrowing the arteries and eventually resulting in atherosclerosis (hardening of the arteries). The antioxidants—vitamin E, vitamin C, and beta-carotene, among others—are thought to have the ability to destroy these free radicals, blocking the oxidation and, as a result, preventing cellular damage and the accumulation of plaque.

By the way, smokers produce much higher amounts of free radicals than nonsmokers. Antioxidants are strongly advised for smokers, although stopping smoking is an even better idea.

"What foods supply these vitamins?"

Good sources of beta-carotene include carrots, dark-green leafy vegetables, parsley, watercress, red bell peppers, sweet potatoes, winter squash, cantaloupe, apricots, and mangoes. Also milk and liver contain significant amounts of vitamin A. Vitamin C comes from citrus fruits, strawberries, kiwifruit, cabbage, parsley, red or green bell peppers, broccoli, cantaloupe, and other produce, while vitamin E is most abundant in vegetable oils, sunflower and other seeds, wheat germ and wheat-germ oil, fortified whole-grain cereals, nuts, and dried beans.

"Is it possible to get enough antioxidants in a balanced daily diet?"

It's extremely doubtful that you could, even if you ate fruits, vegetables, and grains almost exclusively. Most people need supplements to come anywhere near the amounts thought to be protective. The typical daily intake for adults who do not take supplements, for example, is under 10 units of vitamin E. It's even less for those trying to eliminate high-fat foods. To get 100 units from seeds and nuts, you would have to eat two cups of almonds, seven cups of peanuts, or one cup of sunflower seeds. From oils, you would need two cups of corn oil, olive oil, or margarine.

At the same time, remember that the antioxidant theory is still only a hypothesis, although one that seems to provide a key to a simple and safe preventive that could save many lives if it turns out to be correct. And remember, too, that the risks of taking large doses of these vitamins for many years have not yet been established.

"How much of them should I take every day?"

The optimum amounts have not yet been determined, but probably the following daily regimen will do the job: 500 to 1,500 milligrams a day of vitamin C, preferably spaced throughout the day; 400 to 800 units of vitamin E; and 10,000 to 25,000 units of beta-carotene.

"We've all been warned that the saturated fat in butter and meat increases your cholesterol and your chances of having a heart attack and so we switched to margarine as a healthful alternative. Now we learn that the fat in margarine may be even worse. What are we to believe? Even more important, what are we to eat?"

The only answer to this question is to eat less of *all* fats, including butter and margarine. A report by Harvard researchers says that the "trans fatty acids," a new type of fat not found in nature that is created in producing margarine and partially hydrogenated vegetable shortening, may be worse than the saturated fat in butter and meat. Other scientists have questioned these findings, however. In fact, the American Heart Association continues to recommend margarine over butter and prefers soft margarines over the bars because the more liquid in the margarine, the less hydrogenated it is and the less trans fatty acid it contains.

"And what about monounsaturated fats, the kind found in olive oil? They are supposed to be good for you."

Again we don't know for sure but some laboratory research has come up with findings that look promising for "oleate-enriched" oils that are high in monounsaturated fats. Using them along with sufficient vitamin E may help avoid artery clogging in people who have a high risk for CAD.

"Shouldn't everyone take aspirin regularly to prevent heart attacks?"

No—not until it has proven to be helpful and then only with your doctor's approval. On the plus side, a major study at Brigham and Women's Hospital and Harvard Medical School found that aspirin appears to help prevent heart attacks in women as well as men. It reports that women who took from one to six aspirins a week were 25 percent less likely to have a first heart attack than women who took none. And those over 50 did even better—they had a 32 percent reduction in risk. There was no additional preventive benefit for women who took more than that; in fact, for women who took more than fifteen aspirin a week, there was a slight increased risk of brain hemorrhage stroke.

Aspirin has also been found to be successful in preventing second heart attacks. Women who have survived one attack and then start taking it have 52 percent fewer second attacks than those who don't take it. It is also known to benefit those who have had strokes triggered by clots.

However, don't start dosing yourself with aspirin as a preventive before checking with your physician. Aspirin acts as an anticlotting agent, and you must be sure you have no medical condition that precludes its use. Women tend to develop strokes from bleeding into the brain more often than men, and aspirin can aggravate that tendency. Besides, it may give menstruating women heavier periods and cause ulcers to bleed. Studies are under way to explore the risk, benefits, and side effects of aspirin specifically for women.

"How much aspirin is it safe to take on a regular basis?"

If your doctor okays it, a baby aspirin—1¼ grain (or 80 milligrams, a quarter of an adult aspirin)—taken daily is plenty.

"Don't oral contraceptives increase the risk of heart disease?"

No more. Today that is true only for smokers. The new low-dose oral contraceptives are considered safe even in the long term for women up to the age of 50, *if* they don't smoke. In fact, there is some evidence that today's pill may actually be good for your heart because of the estrogen it provides, again if you don't smoke. Oral contraceptives and smoking are a deadly combination. You should also avoid the pill if you suffer from severe hypertension, although it is deemed safe in cases of mild hypertension controlled by medication.

"Does tamoxifen, the hormone given to women to prevent recurrence of breast cancer, reduce the risk of coronary heart disease?"

Probably, although we don't yet know for sure. Swedish researchers, studying 2,365 postmenopausal breast-cancer patients taking part in a randomized trial of tamoxifen, found that women who received the drug for two years had almost one-third fewer hospital admissions for heart disease than a control group; those who took it for five years had almost two-thirds fewer admissions than women who took it for two. On the other hand, tamoxifen may increase the chances of developing uterine cancer.

"I've read that you have more chance of getting a heart attack if you carry most of your weight around your middle. Is this true?"

Where you store your weight is important, according to some studies. Women who gain weight around the middle, as many men do, are at greater risk for heart disease than women with the typically female "pear" shape. Nobody knows why or what you can do about it except to keep your overall weight down.

"How does smoking affect your heart?"

We can best answer that question by telling you that, according to the American Heart Association, smoking is the nation's leading avoidable cause of *all* deaths, including both cardiovascular disease and cancer deaths. Smoking accounts for more than 230,000 deaths from heart and blood-vessel disease a year. And there is an increasing number of studies that link smoking to stroke, particularly the most deadly kind—subarachnoid hemorrhage. One study reports that smokers are three or four times more likely than nonsmokers to have strokes.

The good news is that a year after they kick the habit, former smokers decrease their heart disease risk by more than 50 percent (although this is not true for lung cancer). And within several years, their risk approaches that of people who never smoked.

"I like having a drink before dinner and I've heard that moderate drinking is beneficial to your heart. I think that's wonderful and would like to know the real story."

Alcohol seems to have positive effects on the heart when taken in sensible amounts, and there's been mounting scientific evidence that a drink or two a day can substantially cut the risk of all types of cardiac disease. More than a half-dozen large long-term studies have linked moderate alcohol consumption to 30 to 40 percent less risk of heart attack and coronary heart disease. And the most recent research points to *half* the risk.

The mechanism by which alcohol protects against heart disease probably is that it acts as an antioxidant, preventing LDL cholesterol from clogging coronary arteries and raising the HDL cholesterol that cleanses the blood vessels of fatty buildups. It also seems to have an anticlotting effect, accounting for a reduced risk of stroke in moderate drinkers. The group of researchers recently reported that the highest levels of a naturally occurring enzyme that helps break down clots could be found among those who drank alcohol daily, with the lowest levels among nondrinkers.

A drink or two, however, does not mean a tumbler full of whiskey; in fact, for women, one drink is the definition of moderate. That means 12 ounces of beer, 5 ounces of wine, or 1.5 ounces of 80-proof hard liquor. Each of these drinks contains roughly the same amount of absolute alcohol—about 12 grams.

Heavier drinking actually harms the heart, increasing the risk of coronary disease and hypertension and perhaps, as some studies suggest, breast cancer. In fact, some reports suggest that even moderate alcohol intake may increase the risk of breast and colon cancer. If this contradiction puts you in a quandary, you are not alone.

ALL ABOUT CHOLESTEROL

Because *cholesterol* is one of the major buzzwords of the nineties, you have undoubtedly heard just about as much about it as you ever want to hear. Nevertheless, here are the facts as well as the current proliferating theories.

High blood levels of LDL cholesterol—as well as hypertension and smoking—can play a major part in causing atherosclerosis—thickening and hardening of the arteries, which can lead to heart attacks and strokes. That's because cholesterol and other substances build up in the artery walls, narrowing the blood vessels over time and eventually blocking the normal flow of blood. This process probably starts in childhood, progressing rapidly for some people in their thirties and forties, and becoming threatening for others in their fifties and sixties.

CHOLESTEROL EXPLAINED

Cholesterol is a soft, waxy material produced primarily by the liver that is found in all of the body's cells and is used to manufacture hormones, bile acid, and other essential substances. Transported in the blood by carriers called lipoproteins, cholesterol includes two major fractions: LDL (low-density lipoprotein) and HDL (high-density lipoprotein). LDL, which carries 60 to 80 percent of the body's cholesterol, is used by tissues to build cells, but excessive amounts tend to be deposited in artery walls. HDL's job is to clear cholesterol out of the system by delivering it back to the liver for reprocessing or excretion.

In general, the higher your total cholesterol, the more risk you face of accumulating plaque in your artery walls. A desirable total cholesterol is considered to be below 200 mg/dl (milligrams per deciliter), while a borderline elevated level is from 200 to 240 mg/dl, and a high level is anything above 240 mg/dl.

But total serum cholesterol only hints at the whole picture. What it really means is that, if your level is high, you should be sure to have the cholesterol content analyzed to determine how much of that total is LDL and how much is HDL. And, even better, to determine the ratio of total cholesterol to LDL.

Just to make things more confusing, even if you have a normal total level, you can still have a high proportion of LDL ("bad cholesterol"), which means you are more likely than others to have a heart attack. Or even with a very high total level, you may have a high proportion of HDL ("good cholesterol") and low LDL ("bad cholesterol") which makes the total number meaningless because your elevated HDL renders you less likely to have a heart attack or atherosclerosis. For women, the level of HDL cholesterol is the best predictor of risk.

According to a recent expert panel sponsored by the National Institutes of Health, the likelihood of developing coronary heart disease is greatest among those with HDL levels of less than 35 mg/dl, or those with a total cholesterol-to-HDL ratio greater than 5. It is also considered hazardous if the LDL level is above 170 mg/dl. Many women, especially those with normal levels of estrogen, have elevated totals because they have high HDL levels—just what the doctor ordered because high HDLs protect their arteries.

WHAT THE NUMBERS MEAN

- *Total Cholesterol*
     Under 200 mg/dl: Desirable*
     200 to 240 mg/dl: Borderline*
     Above 240 mg/dl: High*

*Depending on how your cholesterol-to-HDL ratio checks out (see p. 119). Whatever your total cholesterol, you must have your blood analyzed to determine that ratio before you will know if you are safe.

- *High-Density Lipoprotein (HDL)*
    Under 35 mg/dl: Too low
    Between 35 and 60: Borderline
    Above 60 mg/dl: Probably okay, depending on the
    ratio to LDL
- *Low-Density Lipoprotein (LDL)*
    Under 130 mg/dl: Good
    Between 130 and 160 mg/dl: Borderline high
    Above 170 mg/dl: High and hazardous

How to Determine Your Total Cholesterol/HDL Ratio

Divide your total cholesterol number by your HDL number to get the ratio of cholesterol to HDL. The higher the better. If, for example, your total is 300 and your HDL is 22, then your ratio is 13.6. Not good. But if the total measures 300 and your HDL is 90, the ratio comes out at 3.3. That's excellent, despite the high total cholesterol level.

WOMEN AND CHOLESTEROL

Women generally start out with better cholesterol ratios than men, but that changes abruptly at menopause, when their HDL levels tend to drop precipitously and their LDL levels rise. This helps explain the increased risk of coronary artery disease as women get older. But when women take estrogen supplements after menopause, there is little change from premenopausal cholesterol levels because the hormone keeps the HDLs high and the LDLs low. It also keeps the blood vessels more elastic.

"What are triglycerides and are they important?"

Triglycerides are molecules of ordinary fat circulating in the blood and traveling together with cholesterol. Their role in coronary disease remains controversial, but we do know that diabetics who tend to have high triglyceride levels also have an increased risk of plaque-lined arteries and hypertension.

"Do genetics play an important part in cholesterol levels? Both my parents and my brother have high cholesterol and so do I."

Genes are probably the most important reason for abnormally high cholesterol levels, especially when they are accompanied by low HDLs.

"If you don't have hereditary high cholesterol, can you lower your total satisfactorily by diet alone?"

Of course you can, if you work at it hard enough and especially if you combine it with vigorous exercise. Think of all the vegetarians who walk around with cholesterol levels of 140 milligrams.

"I have very high cholesterol, a condition that seems to run in my family, and my doctor wants to put me on a drug that lowers it. Why can't I accomplish the same thing by eating right?"

Because if heart disease runs in your family and you have a genetic tendency to elevated cholesterol, it is extremely unlikely that you can change your situation significantly with diet alone, no matter how strict the diet. Don't get us wrong; it can certainly help to eat a low-fat diet, but it probably won't help enough. When a low-fat diet and weight loss alone don't do the job, cholesterol-lowering drugs are the next step.

"I'd like to raise my HDL to a healthier level. It is usually below 35 mg/dl. What can I do?"

The best way to raise HDL is to exercise regularly. If you're overweight, lose weight. If you smoke, stop. If you are post-menopausal, start taking HRT. Modify your diet. It is not good to have an HDL level that is so low.

HOW TO LOWER YOUR CHOLESTEROL

If you have been told by your physician that it is important for you to lower your cholesterol level, remember that what you want is more HDL and less LDL. Here is the latest prescription:

- *Diet modification.* Eat a low-fat diet, getting the total percentage below 30 percent (the diet of the average American currently derives about 38 percent of calories from fat). Severely limit saturated fats, mainly found in fatty meats, butter, whole milk, cream, eggs, tropical oils, and fats that are solid at room temperature. Avoid polyunsaturated oils such as corn oil that lower serum HDL and substitute monounsaturated oils like olive oil that maintain serum HDL while lowering LDL. Increase your intake of soluble fiber.
- *Garlic.* Eat more garlic, just in case there is truth to the many reports that this member of the onion family lowers cholesterol levels and reduces the risk of heart disease. Researchers at the New York Medical College recom-

mend consuming the equivalent of one-half to one clove of garlic daily, raw or cooked, or taken as deodorized garlic pills. A 600 milligram tablet is equal to about half a fresh clove.

- *Calcium.* Consume sufficient calcium, at least enough to help preserve your bones (see Chapter 4). A high-calcium diet has been linked with higher HDL and lower LDL cholesterol levels.
- *Exercise.* Step up your physical activity. Those who exercise most tend to have lower total cholesterol counts and higher HDLs.
- *Weight control.* Body fat is a major contributor to high cholesterol and coronary risk.
- *HRT.* Discuss hormone replacement therapy with your physician. Women who take HRT boost their HDL levels and lower their LDL.
- *Drug therapy.* If you can't accomplish your goal of raising HDL and/or lowering LDL to acceptable numbers with nondrug measures after a reasonable time, your doctor may recommend one of an increasing array of cholesterol-lowering drugs. All of these have potential for side effects, however, ranging from liver complications to constipation, so their use should be postponed until it has been determined that the dietary regime has failed.

ALL ABOUT HYPERTENSION

High blood pressure, or hypertension, a major risk factor for heart disease and the number one cause of strokes, must be kept under control if you plan to live a long, healthy life. The country's most common chronic illness, hypertension is also one of the most dangerous because almost half the people with hypertension don't know they have it.

FAST FACTS ABOUT HYPERTENSION

- A consistent blood pressure reading of 140/90 is now considered high enough to warrant treatment.
- The prevalence of hypertension increases with age.
- Blood pressure is normally and temporarily raised by exercise and stress. However, regular aerobic exercise lowers overall blood pressure.
- Men have a higher risk of hypertension than women until age 55, when the risk becomes equal.
- Women 65 and older are even more likely than men to develop high blood pressure.
- People with high blood pressure tend to have high cholesterol levels.
- Stress, both physical and mental, causes significantly greater increases in blood pressure among postmenopausal women than it does in either premenopausal women or middle-aged men.

HOW TO LOWER HYPERTENSION

Start off with some changes in lifestyle that may lower your blood pressure enough without resorting to drugs. Even if medication is eventually required, it may be possible to use a lower dose if you practice new habits.

- At the risk of inducing terminal boredom, we must put stopping smoking at the top of the list. This is critical because the combination of smoking and hypertension is particularly deadly.

- Next comes overweight. Losing excessive pounds on a low-fat diet can lower your blood pressure dramatically.
- Decreasing the fat in your diet will automatically increase the fiber because, to get enough to eat, you'll have to consume more fruits and vegetables. That's good, because a Harvard University School of Public Health survey found that men (and undoubtedly women, too) who ate more than 24 grams of fiber per day had a 46 percent lower incidence of high blood pressure than those who consumed less than 12 grams daily.
- Regular aerobic exercise will accomplish the same results.
- Limit your total salt intake to less than 5 grams a day.
- Limit alcohol consumption to a maximum of two drinks a day.
- Increase your calcium consumption to at least 1,000 milligrams a day, the amount you need to build strong bones in any case if you are premenopausal or take HRT. After menopause, without HRT, you need at least 1,500 milligrams a day. There is some evidence that people who have a high level of calcium in their diets have lower blood pressure readings than people whose calcium intake is low, including those with a family history of hypertension. One reason may be that calcium lowers cholesterol levels.
- Eat enough potassium, particularly potassium-rich fruits and vegetables such as bananas, potatoes, winter squash, spinach, and lentils. Evidence has been mounting that hypertension is more prevalent in people who don't consume much of this important mineral, which is easily provided by the average American diet.

HYPERTENSION: THE DRUG ROUTE

If lifestyle changes don't make enough difference in your blood pressure, drug therapy is the next step for protection against strokes, congestive heart failure, kidney disease, and more severe hypertension. Better than 90 percent of hypertensives can be controlled by medication. The drugs commonly used include diuretics, beta-blockers, calcium channel blockers, alpha-blockers, and angiotensin-converting enzyme (ACE) inhibitors.

"How do you know if you have high blood pressure?"

Only by having your blood pressure checked regularly. High blood pressure is known as the silent killer because it usually causes no noticeable symptoms until its most advanced stage, when it has already done most of its damage.

"What's normal and what's high?"

A normal premenopausal woman usually has a blood pressure between 100 over 65 (100/65) and 140 over 90 (140/90). The top number is the systolic pressure, generated each time the heart contracts. The bottom number measures the diastolic pressure, the pressure in the arteries when the heart relaxes between beats. Optimal pressure is below 120/80, but a postmenopausal woman may have a measurement higher than that and still be considered normal because the systolic pressure tends to rise with age as the result of increasing rigidity of the blood vessels.

For all ages, a reading of 140/90 or greater, measured on three consecutive occasions at least a week apart, is generally considered high and cause for concern. A woman with even slightly elevated systolic blood pressure, from 140 to 159, is now considered to be at increased risk of developing both full-fledged hypertension and heart disease.

"My blood pressure goes sky-high when I go to the doctor but it has been normal when I've had it taken in our local pharmacy. How can you explain that?"

That's such a common phenomenon, especially in people over 50, that it's been dubbed "white-coat hypertension." You get so stressed out when you go to the doctor that your blood pressure jumps. It will usually come down if you wait five or ten minutes and have several repeat measurements.

Best to get a home unit and test yourself. To get an accurate measurement, don't smoke for at least a half-hour before the test. Empty your bladder. Sit down and rest for five minutes. Then, in a warm room, apply the cuff to a bare arm. Take two or three readings and average them. In the meantime, consider this phenomenon to be a possible early warning of impending high blood pressure.

"I am 67. My blood pressure seems to skyrocket whenever I am upset or under stress. Is that normal?"

Absolutely, especially for older women. Laboratory tests have found that postmenopausal women have higher blood pressure surges in response to mental stress than either premenopausal women or men of all ages. Researcher C. Noel Bairey, M.D., of Cedars-Sinai Medical Center in Los Angeles, who made the study, suggests daily relaxation therapies such as meditation and yoga that can lower both blood pressure and heart rate, as well as hormone replacement therapy. Regular exercise also helps.

"I want to ask about low *blood pressure rather than hypertension. My blood pressure is usually about 100 over 70. Should I do something about that?"*

On the contrary, you should feel real good about it if you are in good health, because low pressure puts less stress on the blood vessels and increases your chances of a long life.

"My blood pressure medicine doesn't agree with me. It makes me feel dizzy and lightheaded, even nauseated sometimes."

Ask your doctor to change the medication or perhaps to try a lower dose. Sometimes older women do very well on half or even a quarter of the standard dose. Since there are now so many effective medications, the proper dosage and combination can be found for just about everybody.

"Once I start taking drugs, do I have to keep taking them forever?"

Not necessarily. About a third of people who stop drug treatment for hypertension can then maintain normal blood pressure over the long term. But don't quit the medication without your doctor's supervision and be sure to have regular followup tests. The high blood pressure may recur even after you've been off the therapy for many months.

Chapter 6

YOUR BREASTS:
ANSWERS TO YOUR QUESTIONS

WOMEN WORRY MORE ABOUT THEIR BREASTS than any other part of their bodies. Even though they are five times more likely to die of a heart attack, it is breast cancer they fear the most. But the risk of getting breast cancer is a lot less than you probably think. And getting it doesn't mean you're going to die from it because cases picked up early are remarkably curable today.

Most breast problems are not cancer. All breasts have their unique shapes, sizes, lumps, and bumps, and they all change over the years as they respond to fluctuations of hormones and to the passage of time. The vast majority of these variations are perfectly normal. Although they may frighten you at first, most turn out to be common, benign, and no cause for alarm.

WHAT YOU CAN DO *NOW*

The best defense against serious breast problems is to start taking preventive measures as early in your life as possible. For example:

- *Be on the alert.* Start now getting into the habit of paying attention to your breasts. Learn what your breast tissue feels like when it's normal and, if you still have periods, how it changes through your menstrual cycle, so you'll notice any significant changes later on. This means giving yourself a self-exam once a month, seeing the doctor for a breast exam at least once a year, and, most important, having mammography starting at least by age 40, even earlier in some cases. And making an appointment with your doctor whenever you have questions or even the smallest suspicion of a problem.
- *Eat a low-fat, moderate-fiber diet.* Although studies have found no link (except perhaps for vitamin A, which may be helpful) between what you eat and the risk of breast cancer, limiting your fat and consuming more fruits and vegetables keeps you healthier and at lower risk for cancer in general.

  Eat at least one or two servings a day of foods rich in vitamin A. A new study finds that eating less than one daily serving seems to slightly increase your chances of breast cancer. Among the best sources of vitamin A are spinach, carrots, sweet potatoes, cantaloupes, and yellow squash. Some animal foods, like milk and liver, also contain goodly amounts of this vitamin.
- *Limit your consumption of alcoholic drinks.* Don't drink more than a moderate amount. Evidence is accumulating for the potential hazards of alcohol of even one drink every other day. (At the same time, it is mounting for the protective effect of moderate drinking against heart disease!)
- *Get regular exercise.* Studies have found that women who are physically active are at reduced risk for breast cancer.
- *Don't smoke.* A new study by the American Cancer Society reports that a woman's risk of dying from breast cancer increases by 25 percent if she is a smoker. It rises in proportion to the number of cigarettes smoked per day and the number of years she has smoked, culminating with a 75 percent increased risk in women who smoke

two packs a day or more. If you used to be a smoker, relax. The study found no association between former smoking and higher risk.

BENIGN BREAST DISEASE

Benign breast disease (BBD) is the catchall term commonly used to describe all the changes in breast tissue that are *not* malignant. These changes are probably present to some degree in all women, especially over the age of 30, and usually refer to uneveness, bumpiness, thickening, or nodularity, and sometimes discomfort or even pain. They include so many different conditions that all the term BBD really means is that they aren't cancer.

"My breasts get so painful every month that I can't sleep comfortably or even wear my bra. What causes this and what can I do about it?"

Pain is the most common breast symptom women have, but *it is very rarely associated with cancer.* At least half the time, the pain is cyclical, becoming most acute in the week or so before your menstrual period when your body produces high levels of estrogen and progesterone and causes fluid retention and temporary hypertrophy of the mammary glands. Then it is relieved when your period starts and your hormone production bottoms out. Many women find that when their hormone levels start to drop as they get closer to menopause, the discomfort diminishes too.

"I've been told I have fibrocystic breast disease. Is this a serious problem and does it mean I'm going to get breast cancer?"

About half of all women have cystic breasts, a form of benign breast disease so common that it can't be considered a "disease" at all, but simply a variation of normal. It is not a risk factor for breast cancer.

A diagnosis of *fibrocystic breast disease, fibrocystic changes*, or *cystic mastitis* sounds ominous, but it just means you have lumpy breasts. They may become swollen and uncomfortable or even painful, especially just before menstruation, but they are no cause for alarm. The lumpiness is caused by normal hormonal changes, so it and the discomfort come and go with your periods. It most commonly shows up in your thirties or forties, but then improves or vanishes after menopause.

This condition, sometimes in one breast, sometimes in two, is caused by fluid retention and swollen fibrous tissue, which can feel like a thickening ranging in size from that of a small pea to a golf ball. When the fibrous tissue is stretched by hormone-induced fluid collection, the breasts become sore and tender.

Cystic breasts, except for one unusual variation, do not increase your risk of developing cancer. However, because it's sometimes difficult to distinguish between harmless cysts and tumors during a breast exam, regular mammography is important.

Only one kind of cystic or lumpy breasts indicates a higher-than-average risk for breast cancer. That is *atypical hyperplasia*, a premalignant condition with unusual but not specifically cancerous tissue changes. A diagnosis, confirmed by a biopsy, of atypical hyperplasia means you have about four times the normal risk of developing cancer over the next fifteen years, especially if you are premenopausal or have a family history of breast cancer.

HOW TO COPE WITH BREAST TENDERNESS

The best remedies may be the simplest. For starters, avoid caffeine and methylxanthines (coffee, tea, cola, chocolate). In addition, try the following:

- *Vitamins.* Many women swear by vitamin E taken in doses of 400 to 600 units a day. If you add 500 milligrams of vitamin B_6, a natural diuretic, you may find it works even better. There's no scientific evidence to prove the effectiveness of these popular remedies, but it certainly wouldn't hurt to try them to see if they work.
- *Diuretics.* When your breasts are especially tender because of fluid retention and you need more diuretic action than you can get from vitamin B_6, use a commercial diuretic instead when you're feeling symptomatic. Aldactone (spironolactone) is a good choice because it is very mild and can be taken whenever you need it.
- *Low-dose oral contraceptives.* The pill, which blocks ovulation and the cyclical ebb and flow of your hormones, also helps many premenopausal women with breast pain.
- *Prolactin reduction.* Some women tend to make too much prolactin, a breast-stimulating pituitary hormone that sometimes causes breast discomfort. If you prove to have an elevated prolactin level (easily measured by a simple blood test), especially if it is accompanied by galactorrhea (nipple discharge), your doctor may prescribe Parlodel (bromocriptine), a drug that reduces prolactin production.
- *Danazol.* Marketed as Danocrine, this is a weak male hormone that suppresses the breasts' response to estrogen and progesterone, and may also help to relieve the tenderness. It, too, has its side effects—acne, oily skin, water retention, and sometimes irregular vaginal bleeding—and is expensive, but it may be worth a try if nothing else helps.

"What is cystic mastitis? My doctor says it's the reason why my breasts get so painful."

It is simply a more severe variety of fibrocystic breast change, whose symptoms include cysts and fluid retention and also periodic inflammation that is most likely caused by an abnormally sensitive response to a normal level of estrogen or to a higher than normal estrogen level. The usual treatment is aspirin or anti-inflammatory medications such as Advil or Motrin. Sometimes cold packs help, too. In really severe cases, you may have to resort to a few months of treatment with a drug—danazol or Lupron—that shuts off your estrogen production and menstrual periods until the overstimulation and its effects have dissipated.

"Does a diagnosis of fibrocystic breast disease mean I should not take hormones after menopause?"

Although some physicians still warn women away from HRT for this reason, taking hormones will *not* increase your risk of breast cancer. And it is unlikely to cause additional discomfort. The dose of estrogen you get in HRT is so low—much lower than what you used to make when you were younger—that it rarely overstimulates the breast tissue.

If, however, you are among the few women for whom it does cause tenderness, probably because you are unusually sensitive to estrogen, ask your doctor to change the progesterone you take along with the estrogen from the usual kind (Provera) to 19 nor-steroids (Norlutate) before you decide to give up HRT's good effects on your bones and heart. This form of progesterone, with its more androgenic effect, tends to counter estrogen's stimulation of the breasts. For some women, Estratest (a combination of estrogen and low-dose testosterone) accomplishes the same purpose.

If the tenderness persists, you may want to take your HRT cyclically—three weeks on and one week off—rather than every day, which is now the preferred schedule. This way, you'll be receiving a lower total amount of estrogen each month and you will have less breast stimulation.

"Does caffeine cause fibrocystic breasts?"

Neither coffee nor any other form of caffeine is associated with cystic breasts, according to the National Cancer Institute. It can, however, aggravate breast tenderness.

"My breasts are tender all the time. If I don't have cystic breasts, what do I have?"

If you have lumpy breasts with pain that persists and doesn't come and go with your menstrual cycles, you may have *duct ectasia*, a benign condition that is often most troublesome in the years just before and after menopause. This means you have small deposits of calcium in the small clusters of interconnected milk ducts, probably resulting from chronic inflammation.

"The report on my last mammography mentions calcifications. What exactly are they and should I be concerned about them?"

According to the National Cancer Institute, calcifications are small deposits of calcium usually found only by mammography. Most of them are benign. In fact, about half of all women over 50 have coarse calcium deposits called *macrocalcifications*, which are almost invariably nonmalignant. The term *microcalcifications*, on the other hand, refers to smaller more numerous specks of calcium that may be found in an area of rapidly dividing cells. When many of these are seen in one area, they are referred to as a cluster, and may possibly indicate a very early cancer. So when they are detected in a mammogram, they are considered suspicious and must be thoroughly investigated.

"How do you know when the lumps are cysts and not cancer?"

Cysts usually change throughout the menstrual cycle, becoming larger and more uncomfortable just before menstruation. And they are usually quite distinguishable from malignant breast masses because they are round, soft, and movable. Malignant lumps rarely cause pain and rarely change during the cycle. They tend to be harder and more irregular in shape than fibrocystic lumps. Hard lumps that don't move, however, are usually *fibroadenomas*—benign knots of fibrous connective tissue. Nevertheless, they must be investigated.

But don't play doctor. See your physician if you are concerned about what you feel in your breasts. If there is any question, mammography is usually the next step.

Cysts are rarely removed, and their chances of being benign are almost 100 percent. Sometimes they are aspirated in the doctor's office just to prove they are cysts. This means the fluid is drawn out with a very fine needle, temporarily deflating the cyst and providing cells for further examination.

Occasionally, a lump that can be felt with the fingers does not show up in a mammogram, and this is almost always a cyst. In such cases, ultrasound can be used to identify it more accurately.

"How many lumps are malignant?"

We can't answer that question because there are no accurate estimates, but we do know that the percentage is small. Keep in mind that only the lumps that seem suspicious are removed for biopsy. And of all the lumps that are removed because they look suspicious, over 80 percent are found to be harmless.

"What's the difference between benign tumors and malignant tumors?"

Any mass of extra tissue can be benign or malignant. Benign masses are not cancer. They can usually be removed and rarely come back. Their cells do not invade other tissues and do not spread to other parts of the body.

Malignant masses are cancer—abnormal cells that divide without control or order, that can invade and damage nearby tissues and organs through metastasis. This means the cells can break away and enter the bloodstream or lymphatic system, starting secondary tumors in other parts of the body.

"Sometimes I have a slight discharge from my nipples. Should I be concerned about it?"

Nipple discharge (*galactorrhea*) is rarely a serious matter, especially when it occurs in both breasts. Sometimes you'll have milky white discharge after a pregnancy or it may be a side effect of tranquillizers, antidepressants, antianxiety drugs, or certain antihypertensive medications such as Aldomet or reserpine.

A milky discharge may also come from an increase in the pituitary hormone prolactin. In turn, an elevated prolactin level may be caused by low thyroid function or a benign slow-growing tumor of the pituitary gland called a prolactinoma. Taking thyroid hormone corrects the low thyroid function, while a drug marketed as Parlodel (bromocriptine) shrinks the pituitary tumor and stops the breast discharge.

If the discharge is from one breast only, especially if it is bloody, it is usually caused by a benign condition called a *papilloma*. However, it is important to rule out the small possibility of a malignancy.

"What are papillomas?"

Papillomas are tiny growths much like polyps. Found by mammogram or, in some cases, by ductogram (a mammogram taken after dye is injected into a milk duct), they are usually removed because, like colon polyps, they are considered to be a premalignant condition. (By the way, the term *premalignant* means that, left untreated, a condition such as papillomas or polyps could become cancer eventually.)

"My breasts seem to droop more and more every year. Is there anything to do about that?"

No, except to prevent more stretching of the connective tissue by wearing a good supportive bra, especially when you are exercising. Breast tissue loses its elasticity with time, the subcutaneous fat layer decreases, gravity takes its toll, and the fibrous connective tissue diminishes so that they are not as firmly packed or tightly supported as they once were. Some women say estrogen replacement restores some of the elasticity, but that is doubtful. What it may do is cause more breast fullness, thereby making the breasts less flabby.

BREAST CANCER

Although magazine and newspaper headlines insistently announce that one woman in nine will develop breast cancer, the situation is not as bleak as it sounds. Those statistics indicate the *lifetime* accumulated risk that any woman will develop breast cancer between birth and the age of 110. In other words, if you are an average American woman, only if you live to be 110 will your chances be one in nine.

For most of your life, the risk is far lower. For example, the risk between the ages of 35 and 45 is only 1 percent. The risk from birth to 50 is 2 percent; and from birth to age 70 is 6 percent. Not until you reach the age of 95 does your risk reach one in eight.

What all this really means is that, as life expectancy increases among women, we see more breast cancer because it is predominantly a disease of aging. In other words, the older you get, the more likely you are to develop it. This is an important fact to remember because most women seem to consider it a problem that primarily strikes younger women and, therefore, tend not to be on the alert for it as the years pass. As one patient said recently, "I'm seventy-five years old. I don't need to keep on having mammograms. I'm not going to get breast cancer." Wrong.

Extended life expectancy isn't the only reason for an apparent increased incidence of breast cancer in the United States. Another important factor is early detection. Only a few years ago, many cases of breast cancer went undiagnosed and death was attributed to other causes. Now, with mammography more widely used, this disease is identified much earlier, adding to the numbers of reported cases.

No one knows for sure, but the increase could also be attributed to lifelong exposure to rich diets or environmental factors such as cigarette smoke, alcohol, radiation, and toxic chemicals that may cause damage that triggers cancer.

RISK FACTORS FOR BREAST CANCER

Age Just growing older puts you at risk for breast cancer simply because you have lived long enough to get it. Age, in fact, is the major risk factor of all. Two-thirds of cases occur in women over 50 and most breast cancer is diagnosed in women over 65. The reason? One of the conditions specifically required for breast cancer is damage to the DNA inside the cell nucleus. The longer you live, the more cell damage is likely to occur.

Family History The effect of family history is usually overestimated, especially if your relatives developed breast cancer after menopause. Most breast cancers are *not* inherited. Having a mother with breast cancer after the age of 60, for example, gives you no greater risk than having had your first child after age 25. There is significant risk only when a close female relative (mother or sister) had breast cancer *before* menopause, especially before the age of 40, and especially when it affected both breasts. Then the risk is about twice that of other women. If your mother or sister had cancer after 60, however, your risk is increased only slightly; and if she developed it after 80, it's no greater than normal.

Genetic Predisposition Approximately one in 200 women has inherited a defective gene that gives her a heightened susceptibility to breast cancer and puts her at high risk of contracting breast cancer before the age of 50. Scientists are close to pinning down the responsible genetic flaw, also implicated in ovarian cancer, and genetic screening tests will undoubtedly be available within a year or two.

Atypical Hyperplasia   A diagnosis of atypical hyperplasia—a proliferation of abnormal though nonmalignant cells—raises your chances of developing cancer within your lifetime.

Pregnancy   The younger you were at your first pregnancy, the lower your risk of developing breast cancer later in life. Conversely, women who delay childbirth until after 30 or who remain childless have a greater chance of getting it.

Breastfeeding   You will have a 46 percent lower risk of getting breast cancer *before* menopause if you started breastfeeding before the age of 20 and continued for at least six months. However, early breastfeeding seems to have no effect on your chances of developing it *after* menopause.

Menstruation   The age you had your first period and the age you had your last has a small effect on your risk of breast cancer. If you began to menstruate before the age of 12 or began your menopause after age 55, your chances are minimally elevated. And just the opposite, if you menstruated at a later age and reached menopause earlier than usual, thus having a lower lifetime level of estrogen, you will tend to have a slightly lower risk of breast cancer.

The Warning Signs

- A lump or a thickening in the breast. This is the most common warning sign of cancer, although almost all lumps turn out to be benign.
- A change in the shape or contour of your breast, including the nipple and the area (areola) around it.

- A bloody discharge from the nipple (again, usually benign).
- A change in the color or texture of the skin, such as a dimpling or puckering.
- An inverted or retracted nipple, if it wasn't present before.
- Hard swollen lymph glands in the armpit.

THE IMPORTANCE OF EARLY DETECTION

Getting breast cancer doesn't mean dying from breast cancer. Detected early, when it is still very small and hasn't invaded the surrounding tissue, breast cancer can be cured at least 90 percent of the time. The only way it can be found so early is by mammography.

It takes a single malignant cell about ten years to reach a size that can be felt with the fingers of the most skilled physician, and most breast cancers aren't discovered until they have been growing about twelve years. With mammography, however, it's possible to find a cancer that's been growing only about seven years and is still too miniscule to be felt by hand. Although there are other kinds of breast-imaging techniques used to detect cancer, such as ultrasound, thermography, and magnetic resonance imaging, mammography is the most effective by far.

That's why every woman over the age of 40 (and earlier in some cases)—despite recent reports that recommend a starting age of 50—should have regular mammography, especially when there are suspicions of problems. Fewer than a third of American women are currently screened as often as necessary, particularly older women who need it the most.

In fact, the older a woman becomes, the less likely she is to have mammography. The National Cancer Institute reported in 1988 that 62 percent of American women over 40 had never had a mammogram, and that only 6.5 percent had had a mammogram in the last year. Older women, those over 60, were particularly negligent about being tested, even though they are the ones who are at a higher risk of developing breast cancer.

Breast Surveillance Guidelines

Although there is controversy concerning the value of mammograms for women under 50, we strongly recommend starting by age 40. When the best equipment is used and the X-ray pictures are interpreted by skilled radiologists, many early cancers are picked up in women still in their thirties and many more among those in their forties. Therefore, we recommend the following guidelines:

If you are under 40

- Examine your breasts every month.
- Have a breast exam by your doctor every year.
- Have your first mammogram between the ages of 35 and 40.

If you are between 40 and 45

- Examine your breasts every month.
- Have a breast exam by your doctor every year.
- Have a mammogram every two years.

If you are 45 or over

- Examine your breasts every month.

- Have a breast exam by your doctor every year.
- Have a mammogram every year.

"What's the best way to go about examining your own breasts?"

The purpose of self-examination is to become familiar with your breasts so you will notice any changes from one month to another. The technique you use isn't as important as making sure you do it at least once a month, two or three days after your periods end if you still have them or at the same time every month, such as the first day of the month, if you don't.

Here is the method for self-examination recommended by the National Cancer Institute.

1. Stand in front of a mirror. Inspect both breasts for anything unusual.
2. Watching closely in the mirror, clasp your hands behind your head and press your hands forward, feeling your chest muscles tighten. Look for any change in the shape or contour of your breasts.

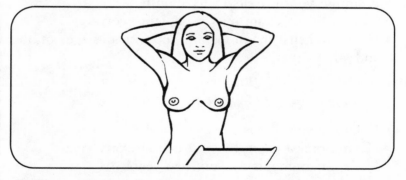

3. Next, press your hands firmly on your hips and bow slightly toward your mirror as you pull your shoulders and elbows forward. Again, look for changes in shape.

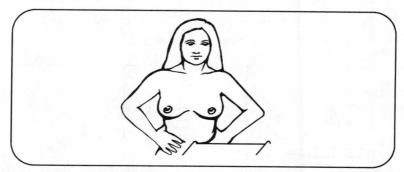

4. Some women do the next part of the exam in the shower because fingers glide over soapy skin, making it easy to concentrate on the texture underneath. Raise your left arm. Use three or four fingers of your right hand to explore your left breast firmly, carefully, and thoroughly. Beginning at the outer edge, press the flat part of your fingers in small circles, moving the circles slowly around the breast. Gradually work toward the nipple. Be sure to cover the entire breast. Pay special attention to the area between the breast and the underarm, including the underarm itself. Feel for any unusual lump or mass under the skin.

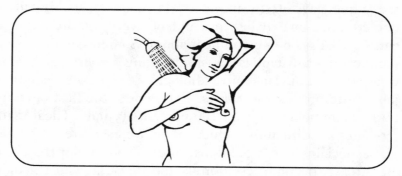

5. Gently squeeze the nipple and look for a discharge. Repeat steps 4 and 5 on your right breast.

6. Steps 4 and 5 should be repeated lying down. Lie flat on your back with your left arm over your head and a pillow or folded towel under your left shoulder. This position flattens the breast and makes it easier to examine. Use the same circular motion described earlier. Repeat the exam on your right breast.

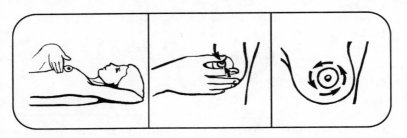

Remember that self-examination, although essential, is not a substitute for routine mammograms or yearly breast exams by a doctor. If you notice any changes, however, see your doctor as soon as you can. Don't panic. Remember that most breast changes are nothing to worry about.

"Don't mammograms make mistakes sometimes? I've heard of women who had breast cancer that mammography didn't pick up."

Mammography isn't perfect, although the equipment and the technique have vastly improved in recent years. It fails to detect about one malignancy out of every hundred and, of course, that's the one you hear about. Sometimes the equipment used is substandard or isn't working properly, and sometimes the technicians and radiologists don't do an adequate job of interpreting the X-rays. Even under the best of conditions, mammography isn't 100 percent accurate. Clear mammograms are difficult to achieve if your breasts are very dense and especially if they are dense and you are under the age of 50. Breasts become less fibrous and dense as you get older and so become easier to examine.

"How can I find a reliable facility for mammography?"

Make sure the facility you are considering has been accredited by the American College of Radiology (ACR) and/or certified by the FDA. This means that the equipment, personnel, and procedures have been evaluated and approved. Accuracy is affected by the skill of the technologist who takes the pictures, the proficiency of the radiologist who interprets them, and how well the X-ray equipment is calibrated.

For More Information

The American College of Radiology provides an updated list of its accredited facilities to the National Cancer Institute each month. For accredited establishments in your area, call: the Cancer Information Service, 1-800-4-CANCER; or the American Cancer Society, 1-800-ACS-2345. Or call 1-800-358-9295 for a copy of the FDA's new guidelines for mammography.

Not all high-quality facilities have been accredited yet, although they may have applied for accreditation. If the one you are considering is among them, check it out by asking these questions before you make an appointment:

1. Does the facility use dedicated mammography machines that have been specifically designed for breast screening?
2. Is the person who takes the mammograms a registered technologist who has been certified by the American Registry of Radiological Technologists or licensed by the state?
3. Is the radiologist who reads the mammograms board-certified and has he or she taken special courses in mammography?
4. Does the facility provide mammograms as part of its regular practice and does it perform at least ten mammograms a week?

5. Is the mammography machine calibrated at least once a year to be sure its measurements and doses are correct?

MAMMOGRAPHY: WHO NEEDS IT?

A mammogram is an X-ray picture of the breast that can pick up clusters or lumps of abnormal cells too small to be detected by touch. It works by pinpointing microcalcifications—tiny deposits of calcium that may be an early sign of cancer.

For a mammogram, you are asked to undress above the waist. Then a technologist positions each of your breasts, one at a time, between two plastic plates that compress it, spreading it out to produce as precise an image as possible. Usually, two views of each breast are taken, one from the side and· one from above. Sometimes additional views are necessary when, for example, the pictures are imperfect, or the view is obscured by dense tissue, or the radiologist wants to take a closer look at a specific area.

Some women find the procedure uncomfortable because of the compression required for a clear picture, but it is rarely painful and lasts only a few seconds. If you are still menstruating, schedule the mammography just after the end of your period, when your breasts are least likely to be tender. The entire mammography procedure lasts about fifteen minutes.

The radiologist, a physician who has been specially trained to read X-rays, studies the photographs and reports the findings to you or your physician.

"Who needs mammography?"

You, at least after you've reached 40. And you probably should start regular mammograms earlier than that if you have a strong family history of breast cancer, if there are any warning signs, or if your breasts are especially heavy and/or dense and therefore difficult to examine thoroughly by palpation.

Mammography is so safe today that there is no downside to it. It won't harm you and it could save your life.

"How often should I have mammography? It's expensive and I don't want to expose myself to too much radiation, either."

The recommendation of the experts is that all women should have a baseline mammography between the ages of 35 and 40 to use for comparison with later pictures. From 40 to 45, you should schedule a mammogram every two years and see your physician once a year for a breast examination. Over the age of 45, mammograms and breast examinations should be scheduled every year.

That's the recommended schedule for women with no symptoms or high risk. If you've had suspicious warning signs or you have a strong family history of breast cancer, talk to your doctor about the wisdom of more frequent mammograms.

A mammogram usually costs anywhere from $75 to $250 and is usually at least partially covered by health insurance, including Medicare. If you are not covered by health insurance, check out the free or low-cost mammography offered by many health agencies and women's support groups. It is best, however, to avoid portable X-ray machines because they tend not to be as accurate as those in established locations.

"I worry about all that radiation. I've heard it's dangerous. Can the radiation from a mammography give you breast cancer?"

Stop worrying. Modern mammography is safe. It uses such a low dose of radiation that there is virtually no risk from the procedure itself. In fact, you would receive an equivalent amount of radiation if you lived in Denver for a year or flew in an airplane for half an hour. Another way of putting it is that the risk of dying of breast cancer caused by one mammogram is the same as that of dying from lung cancer after smoking one cigarette. In any case, the benefits far outweigh any possible risk.

"I've had breast implants. Do they make it harder to read mammograms accurately?"

There has been growing concern that silicone breast implants (augmentation mammaplasty) can make it more difficult to interpret mammography, especially when the scar tissue around the implant thickens and contracts.

On the other hand, most good radiologists have now had considerable experience with implants and have learned new techniques such as displacement mammography and additional views for getting the best results.

"Are there any drawbacks to starting mammograms in my thirties?"

One drawback is that mammograms in younger women with dense breasts tend to set off false alarms, requiring needless fear and unnecessary biopsies to check anomalies that ultimately turn out not to be cancer. Another is that many suspicious-looking abnormalities eventually go away by themselves. And, finally, mammograms cost money.

"And in my forties?"

By then, the incidence of breast cancer has started to increase and many lives could be saved with screening. The only downside for this age group is cost.

"Why can't an MRI—magnetic resonance imaging—be used for detection of malignancies?"

A new development is the magnetic resonance mammogram (MRM) that is currently being tested at several medical institutions, including New York University Medical Center. To date, the MRM has been found to be extremely accurate in detecting cancers (not 100 percent, of course), although very expensive.

"I haven't had a mammogram because I've heard it's very painful. I'd rather take my chances."

Many women avoid having mammograms for the same reason but, in a recent British survey of 600 women who had just had their first mammograms, two-thirds of the women said it was not as uncomfortable as they had anticipated and only 6 percent said it was painful. In a larger study in the United States, 90 percent either had no complaint or felt only mild discomfort. Just 1 percent called the test painful.

But, even if having a mammogram turns out to be uncomfortable for you, remember it takes only a few seconds. Schedule your appointment for a week or so after the start of your period, if you are still menstruating, because that's when your breasts tend to be least tender.

"My radiology laboratory told me not to use deodorant, body powder, or lotions before my mammography. Why?"

Because sometimes they cause confusing shadows on the film.

"What happens when a lump is found?"

When a lump is thought to be merely a harmless cyst, the doctor may order additional mammogram views and/or an ultrasound examination, which uses high-frequency sound waves to produce an image of the interior of the breast and can usually help distinguish between a solid mass and a fluid-filled cyst. The newest technique involves high-resolution digital ultrasound, which improves the ability to make accurate distinctions and reduces the need for biopsies.

Or the doctor may perform a simple needle aspiration right there in the office. With only a local anesthetic, the lump is punctured with a very fine needle and the fluid or a small amount of tissue is withdrawn from it. If it is found to be a fluid-filled cyst, it is not cancer. If it is a solid mass, it is considered suspect and so the sample must go to a laboratory to be checked out.

Another alternative is a tissue biopsy. When the mass is solid, the doctor, usually a surgeon, cuts out part or all of it through a small skin incision under a general anesthesia. The tissue is then sent to a pathologist, who examines it under a microscope for abnormal cells.

A relatively new biopsy technique—stereotactic breast biopsy—is now being used in a growing number of medical institutions to help diagnose very tiny microcalcifications that are deep inside the breast where they cannot be felt but have been detected by mammography. Guided by a special stereoscopic X-ray machine that provides a three-dimensional view of the lump, a spring-loaded "gun" shoots a hollow-core needle into the lesion and extracts a core of tissue to be examined by a pathologist.

DON'T PANIC

Don't panic if your doctor decides to perform a biopsy. Four out of five lumps or suspicious findings turn out to be benign. And there's no need to worry either that you'll wake up from the anesthesia to find you've had your breast removed. Those days are over. Today, even when the lump is found to be malignant, you will be given time for consultations and second opinions before any further steps are taken.

"How is breast cancer treated?"

There are four standard ways to treat breast cancer: surgery, radiation, chemotherapy, and hormone therapy.

Surgery may be lumpectomy, when only the mass and some of the surrounding normal tissue are removed. Or it may be mastectomy, which today need not be drastic. In most cases, surgeons perform a partial mastectomy; a simple mastectomy (removal of the breast but not of the chest muscles); or a modified radical mastectomy, when the breast is removed along with axillary lymph nodes in the armpit but leaves the underlying chest muscles largely intact.

Radiation therapy is the administration of high-energy rays that kill off cancer cells that may have been left behind. Usually used after lumpectomy, it is begun a week or two following the surgery and is usually given five days a week and continued for five or six weeks. It can be applied externally by a radiation machine or internally via radioactive implants.

Chemotherapy is the use of drugs to kill cancer cells. The drugs are given by mouth or by injection into a vein or muscle and travel to all parts of the body through the bloodstream. They are taken in cycles, with recovery periods between treatments.

Hormone therapy treats the cancer by removing, blocking, or adding hormones. Sometimes drugs are used to block the hormones that nourish some breast cancers. Sometimes the ovaries that produce the female hormones are surgically removed. And sometimes hormones are added to fight the cancer.

The most common form of hormone therapy today is tamoxifen (Nolvadex), a hormone itself that competes in certain areas with the body's own estrogen without blocking its production. It is used to fight breast cancers that have been found to be estrogen-dependent—in other words, cancers that require estrogen for growth.

BREAKING NEWS

Taxol, a new drug first derived only from the bark of the Pacific yew tree but now available in synthetic form, may prove to be an effective treatment for breast cancer as well as ovarian cancer, and there have been some encouraging preliminary results. Clinical trials have confirmed that it can shrink ovarian tumors by at least one half in 20 to 30 percent of patients.

Retinoic acid, a derivative of vitamin A, may also become a useful drug for combating breast cancer, but clinical trials have not yet begun in the United States.

WHAT CAUSES BREAST CANCER?

Nobody knows what causes breast cancer, although we know there are certain risk factors that increase the chances of developing it. We know it isn't contagious and it isn't caused by bumps and bruises. And the preponderance of evidence shows little or no association between hormone replacement therapy and increased breast-cancer risk. Current thinking is that a defective gene, sometimes inherited, sometimes caused by damage during a lifetime, may prove to be the biological "master switch" that can trigger breast cancer.

"I've heard that eating a high-fat diet, especially animal fat, will trigger breast cancer. Is this true?"

So far, there is no hard evidence of a correlation between the level of fat consumption and breast cancer. Because American women get breast cancer at a rate five times greater than Japanese women, there has been considerable speculation about the effect of diet on breasts. The prime suspect has been dietary fat, but to date no studies have shown a solid link between the two, nor does there seem to be any protection provided by a low-fat diet except, perhaps, among women who have had a limited fat intake, perhaps even a vegetarian diet, since they were very young children.

So our point of view is that, although there are many good reasons for limiting fat, especially animal fat, preventing breast cancer does not seem to be one of them. Some studies suggest that eating plenty of fruits and vegetables, especially those containing vitamins A, C, and E—the antioxidants—and getting plenty of exercise may provide some protection. Whether they do or not, they certainly can't hurt, and they may well reduce your risk of other problems such as cardiovascular disease and colon cancer.

"What about alcohol? Don't women who drink have a higher incidence of this kind of cancer?"

Just one or two alcoholic drinks a day, studies have found, are enough to put women at a *slightly* greater risk of developing breast cancer.

Some experts think that the younger you were when you started drinking and the greater the number of alcoholic drinks you consume per week, the higher your risk. If this is true, the answer may lie in the poor nutrition or other lifestyle factors usually associated with alcohol abuse.

"Is it true that regular exercise decreases your chances of breast cancer?"

Women who were college athletes, women who work in physically demanding jobs, and women who exercise regularly have decreased breast-cancer rates—the result, some researchers believe, of lower estrogen levels. Women who exercise usually have more lean muscle tissue and less fat tissue than women who don't exercise, and leaner women tend to produce less estrogen. Of course, people who exercise regularly also tend to have other healthy habits, like eating well and not smoking, which may be the reason for their reduced risk.

"Isn't exposure to certain chemicals supposed to cause many kinds of cancer?"

Yes and, in fact, a new study by researchers at the Mount Sinai School of Medicine in New York City shows that women with the highest exposure to the pesticide DDT have four times the breast-cancer risk of women with the least exposure. Although DDT was phased out in 1972 in the United States, most Americans still carry the residues stored in their bodies and the pesticide is still widely used in other countries. Other pollutants in air, water, and food may be linked to breast cancer too, and some are about to be studied by the EPA. These include several pesticides such as endosulfan, DDT, dioxin, and PCBs.

"Do oral contraceptives cause breast cancer?"

No, according to a recent study of nearly 10,000 women, not even among women who have a family history of this disease. And in a recent review of over forty major studies, the Institute of Medicine of the National Academy of Sciences found no increased risk of breast cancer in women ages 20 to 54 who have taken birth-control pills over those who have never used them.

There's one catch. Although oral contraceptives have been available for thirty years and are probably the most studied drug in history, we still don't know their effect on women over the age of 60, when most breast cancer occurs. The likelihood, however, is that the use of low-dose hormones in the pill actually *decreases* the risk for older women.

"Does estrogen cause breast cancer?"

No, estrogen does not cause breast cancer. It can, however, accelerate the growth of some cancers that already exist. However, the prognosis for women who have breast cancer while taking estrogen replacement is much better than for those not taking it, according to a recent Swedish epidemiological study. The reason may be that, although estrogen speeds the growth of the cancer, it does not make it more malignant.

Meanwhile, the tumor is found more readily at a stage when it has not invaded the surrounding tissues.

"So why are women with breast cancer treated with drugs that block their estrogen?"

Because some breast cancers are estrogen-dependent, which means they will grow when they are stimulated by estrogen. Others are not. It is absolutely essential to determine whether an existing malignancy is or is not dependent on estrogen, a fact that can be established by sophisticated hormone-receptor tests. Supplemental estrogen shouldn't be given to anyone with an existing estrogen-dependent cancer, because, although it was not responsible for initiating it, it can make this kind of cancer grow more rapidly. That's why the ovaries may be removed and estrogen blockers prescribed to starve any undiscovered cancer cells.

"There have been recent reports that hormone replacement therapy can cause breast cancer. I am taking estrogen for lots of good reasons, including the prevention of osteoporosis and heart disease, and now I'm worried that it's going to give me breast cancer."

There's been plenty of controversy about this subject and considerable panic among users of hormone replacement therapy because some epidemiologists have suggested that hormone replacement increases the risk of breast cancer. But we don't believe this is true. Although some European studies have suggested a slightly increased incidence after fifteen years on estrogen, most American studies have found no increase at all.

Indeed, some researchers present data suggesting that HRT may actually help to prevent breast cancer. Our own twenty-two-year prospective double-blind study, for example, came up with a lower risk rate for women on hormone replacement. After the first ten years, the incidence of breast cancer in a control group of women who took no hormones was 4.8 percent, while no cancers were found in a group on estrogen replacement. After twelve more years, the incidence in women who had never taken HRT was 11.5 percent, while the incidence among those who had ever taken estrogen supplements remained at zero.

The Women's Health Initiative, a fourteen-year study sponsored by the National Institutes of Health designed to track the health and dietary habits of hundreds of thousands of postmenopausal women, will eventually provide even more answers to the questions about HRT.

"So why do some doctors readily prescribe hormones and others don't?"

HRT must be carefully explained and individualized, and that takes a lot of a doctor's time. Sometimes busy physicians, especially those in primary care, take the easy way out and either prescribe one standard therapy for all of their female patients or none. And sometimes they have little experience in this field.

But virtually all gynecologists and endocrinologists who treat menopausal women every day and remain current on all of the newest research now believe that HRT, while it must not be dispensed indiscriminately, should be seriously considered for every woman at menopause. Even if we believed (which we do not) that HRT causes an increased risk of breast cancer, we think its benefits far outweigh the risk except in rare cases. Heart disease and osteoporosis are both much more likely to kill or disable you than breast cancer.

"I had breast cancer eleven years ago. The doctors say I am cured. Can I go on estrogen?"

You may be cured, but you still run a higher risk than other women of developing new breast cancer. So because estrogen makes breast cancer grow faster although it does not cause it, we recommend hormone replacement only if you need it badly to protect your bones. Have your bones measured and, if they show a dangerous loss, HRT would probably be worth the risk because osteoporosis can kill you, too. But you must have your breasts checked out regularly. And, for you, although the FDA may not concur, we recommend mammograms twice a year.

If your bones are not in serious danger but you need estrogen because intercourse has become painful, there's some really good news. We have found that only 1 gram of conjugated estrogen vaginal cream, inserted in the vagina once a week, will help recornify (thicken) the vagina and make it dramatically more functional. This tiny amount of hormone (the usual dose is 4 grams three times a week) has been found not to be absorbed into the bloodstream and therefore will not affect your risk of cancer. To be absolutely sure, however, your blood estrogen levels should be checked every so often.

Another possibility is a form of progesterone called megesterol (Megace), the only progesterone approved by the FDA for breast-cancer patients. It can give some relief for hot flashes, dry vagina, and the other typical symptoms of estrogen deprivation (see Chapter 7).

"My mother had breast cancer. So should I avoid hormones? I have severe hot flashes and palpitations and, being small-boned, I worry about osteoporosis. How do I solve my dilemma?"

You have twice the normal chance of developing breast cancer in your lifetime if your mother or sister had it before menopause. However, the risk is not high enough, in our opinion, to deprive yourself of the benefits of HRT. Of course, you must be sure to have regular mammography.

"Do silicone implants cause breast cancer? Should I have mine removed as a precaution?"

There has been absolutely no indication that implants cause cancer. There's growing concern, however, that they may be linked with immune disease problems such as lupus and connective tissue diseases such as arthritis or scleroderma, although, after studying almost three decades of medical records of 749 women with implants, scientists at the Mayo Clinic failed to find an association between implants and these diseases.

If you have implants, your doctor will probably test your ANA (antinuclear antibodies) once a year. If the ANA test is positive, there may be a silicone leak that can usually be verified by feel or mammogram. Obviously, a leaky implant should be removed.

TAMOXIFEN: A DREAM DRUG?

If you examine yourself regularly and have mammograms every year, it is a virtual certainty that any cancer that develops will be found early enough for a cure. But there is hope on the horizon that tamoxifen (Nolvadex), a synthetic hormone that blocks the effects of estrogen on breast tissue, may prove to be a dream drug that can fend off cancer before it even begins. It may prevent the minuscule biological changes in the cells that cause the disease.

Tamoxifen has been used for about twenty years as a treatment for advanced breast cancer and, more recently, as an additional therapy along with radiation and chemotherapy for early estrogen-dependent malignancies. It helps prevent recurrence of existing cancer or the development of new cancer and is often given for five to ten years.

Tamoxifen is a weak estrogen, competing with estrogen for receptor sites on the cancer cells and preventing it from getting into the tumor cells, thereby depriving them of the fuel they may need for growth.

This powerful drug may turn out to be a lifesaver, but we won't know for sure until the results come in from an important five-year double-blind study, coordinated by the government's National Cancer Institute, that began late in 1992. The study is investigating the effectiveness of long-term tamoxifen therapy in preventing invasive breast cancer in 16,000 healthy American women who have increased risk for the disease. This group includes women over 60, women with family histories of breast cancer, and women who have had suspicious breast lumps in the past. A similar large-scale trial of tamoxifen is under way in Great Britain.

The hope is that tamoxifen may halt cancer at a stage when biochemical changes have already occurred but before the tumors can be detected by mammography or physical examination. On the other hand, there is concern about the possible hazards of exposing healthy women to so many years of treatment by this powerful drug. In addition to causing especially severe menopausal symptoms like hot flashes and a racing pulse, its possible dangers include liver damage, eye damage, and an increased threat of blood clots. It also has been accused of causing a heightened risk of uterine cancer.

"Isn't tamoxifen supposed to prevent osteoporosis, just like estrogen? And what about coronary heart disease?"

Tamoxifen seems to be similar to estrogen in its ability to prevent osteoporosis by increasing bone density. So that's one thing breast-cancer patients won't have to worry about when they take this drug to block their estrogen. It has also been found to lower total cholesterol and LDL levels—just what the doctor ordered. What it won't do is suppress hot flashes or the unpleasant effects of menopause on your vagina and therefore your sex life.

"I have heard that taking supplementary selenium will help prevent breast cancer. How much should I take?"

We suggest you take none. There is no scientific basis for considering a low level of this element to be a risk factor.

Although some studies have shown lower blood selenium levels among breast-cancer patients, these levels vary hour by hour according to your diet and so don't reflect long-term exposure.

BREAST IMPLANTS

About 2 million American women have had breast implants, about a million of them silicone, in the thirty years that they have been available, but only recently have there been questions about their long-term safety. In 1992, the Food and Drug Administration, responding to growing concern about a possible link between silicone implants and connective-tissue disease, removed this kind of implant from the marketplace until further research proves its safety. Implants filled with saline solution (salt water) remain available, although they, too, are being investigated.

Chapter 7

SEX: WHAT A WOMAN OVER 40 NEEDS TO KNOW

NOT SO LONG AGO, their sexual proclivities and problems were subjects women rarely discussed with anybody, including their doctors, but today women have little hesitation about facing the facts of sexual life and are much more open about their sexuality. What most concerns women over 40? Their libidos and their dry vaginas.

Will diminishing hormones dim your desire and limit your ability to have good sex? The truth is they certainly can, unless you know the part they play and what you can do to avoid, prevent, or correct potential problems.

If you are around 40, just when you've reached the peak of your sexuality you are also perimenopausal or closing in on it—in the United States, the mean age for menopause is 52 years. If you are around 50 and especially if you are older than that, you are undoubtedly already experiencing at least some of the effects of estrogen (and androgen) deprivation. How those effects can alter your sexual interest and activity depends on your health, your "biological age," your attitude, your doctor, and the choices you make.

WHAT YOU CAN DO *NOW*

There's much you can do to prevent pleasurable sexual encounters from turning into painful experiences if you remember that estrogen, the primary female hormone, was responsible for preparing your body at puberty for the possibility of childbearing. Now, after decades of fertility, your estrogen level is falling, turning off the intricate mechanisms that kept your reproductive organs in peak operating condition. As it gradually diminishes, many physical changes take place internally and externally, all of them becoming progressively more pronounced with each passing year. If there ever was a good time to give your vagina some serious consideration, it is now.

- *Schedule a thorough evaluation.* Have a checkup of your vaginal health, whether or not you see signs of impending menopause or are suffering from menopausal symptoms. Do the same no matter how far beyond menopause you are. If sex has already become uncomfortable, it's especially important to see your doctor and talk openly about what you can do about it.
- *Don't give up sex.* Sexually active women maintain vaginal health much better and longer than those who don't.
- *Use a lubricant.* Apply a lubricant before sexual intercourse to ease the effects of a drying vagina.
- *Use a vaginal moisturizer.* This will replenish the tissues.
- *Before menopause, consider going on the pill.* The newest low-dose combination kind (see Chapters 2 and 9) not only prevents pregnancy and regulates erratic periods but helps keep your vagina lubricated and elastic.
- *After menopause, consider going on HRT.* This is a good idea for all the reasons discussed below.

WHAT'S HAPPENING TO YOUR VAGINA

Let's get to the bad news first, the fact that the atrophic changes that can eventually make sexual intercourse extremely uncomfortable, perhaps painful, maybe even impossible, are inevitable if you do nothing about them. Then we will discuss all the ways to practice preventive maintenance for the vagina and get around those problems. Here's what's going on inside of you:

THE BAD NEWS

- *Blood flow.* Without the stimulation of once-abundant estrogen, the blood flow to the genitals gradually declines.
- *Cells.* Cell growth and multiplication decrease since estrogen acts as a growth stimulant on cells.
- *New dimensions.* The size, shape, and flexibility of the vagina changes. It becomes dryer, narrower, less pliable and expandable, maybe even a little shorter, all of which can definitely hinder your ability to enjoy sex. Without estrogen stimulation, its lining loses its tough outer layer of protective cornified cells and becomes thinner, smoother, less elastic, and more easily irritated. It also loses its rugal folds, the thick cushiony folds that allowed for elasticity and expansion. As a result, you may experience not only dry vagina that can dampen your ardor but real pain.
- *Arousal.* It takes longer to become sexually aroused and longer as well to produce lubrication in preparation for intercourse.
- *Dryness.* Lubrication, usually the first noticeable sign of depleted estrogen, gradually decreases as the quantity of secretions slows down. Obviously, a vagina that is dry and unlubricated can be a deterrent to sexual enjoyment. If it isn't moist enough, the penis rubs against sensitive

tissues and causes abrasions that may become inflamed. If you lose estrogen very gradually and/or continue to produce more in both the ovaries and your fat tissue for many years, you won't find dryness a problem at first, but you certainly will eventually.

- *Change in pH.* The vagina becomes more alkaline. A more alkaline pH combined with the new fragility of the vaginal lining makes it much more susceptible to infections than it ever was before. The higher pH level encourages the invasion of contaminate bacteria that cause vaginal infections, while at the same time it discourages the normal organisms that serve to protect you from them.
- *Urethra.* The tissue of the urethra, right next door to the vagina, becomes thinner, more fragile, more likely to be traumatized during intercourse, and more hospitable to the invasion of unfriendly organisms which it may pass along to the vagina. Both the vagina and the urethra (as well as the bladder) are estrogen-dependent organs.
- *Sensory perception.* The ability to feel and respond to touch diminishes with the lack of estrogen.
- *Other signs.* Pubic hair becomes less abundant, the external genitalia lose fatty tissue and flatten, and the clitoris shrinks.

AGONY OR ECSTASY?

It is all of those atrophic physiological responses to estrogen deficiency that can affect your attitude toward making love because all of them take you farther down the road to *dyspareunia*, or painful sex. In addition to the friction from insertion and penetration, you may suffer from itching, burning, pressure, and postcoital bleeding. And these difficulties, if not treated, can lead to other kinds of dysfunctions that include a loss of sexual desire. After all, who looks forward to sex that hurts?

So, unless you want to give up sexual intercourse because

it has become unpleasant, there are steps that must be taken. Although you may be among those fortunate women who continue to manufacture enough estrogen throughout their lives to keep their tissues functioning adequately for a long time, you can't escape the vaginal symptoms forever. And it is virtually certain that you will have to give up pleasurable sexual intercourse eventually, *unless* you replace the estrogen you once made.

What's Your Timetable?

Although some women start encountering difficulties with dry vaginas and the other uncomfortable changes several years before menopause, the problems usually begin after your menstrual periods have stopped. Some women complain of vaginal problems only six months after menopause, especially after a surgical menopause, while for others it may take five or ten years before uncomfortable intercourse becomes routine.

HORMONES AND YOUR SEX DRIVE

The depletion of estrogen in midlife doesn't seem to affect sexual desire and orgasmic ability one way or the other for most women as long as intercourse remains comfortable. Psychologically, some women find their interest in sex grows as their early inhibitions vanish along with the demands of children and the fear of pregnancy. And, physically, libido may even increase as naturally produced male hormones, previously overshadowed by estrogen, become more influential.

Other women lose interest, some because the physical

changes can certainly take their toll, others because they never cared much for sex anyway, or consider it an activity better suited to the young. Maybe more important, they may not have a partner who turns them on. The best stimulus to sexual interest is an ardent lover.

But sometimes the problem of a waning libido can be attributed to a decrease in *androgens*, the male hormones that all women produce in their ovaries along with the female kind. Androgens were once considered exclusively male, but most experts today believe that one of them, testosterone, is the libido hormone for both men and women. Men produce perhaps ten times as much testosterone as women, but this androgen is thought to play an important part in fueling the sex drive in women, too. According to psychiatrist Helen Singer Kaplan, M.D., director of the Human Sexuality Program at the New York Hospital-Cornell Medical Center, "Testosterone is as important to women as it is to men in order to have full libido."

If both of your ovaries are removed or severely damaged, you promptly lose almost all of your androgen production (a small amount is produced by the adrenal glands) and, as a result, may suffer a dramatic loss of interest in sex along with a loss of sensation and may have difficulty achieving an orgasm. Even with a natural menopause, the production of testosterone decreases by nearly 50 percent, although the ovaries usually continue to secrete some androgens for many years.

What to do about that? You can be tested for testosterone and, if your level is very low, a small amount can be taken alone or combined with estrogen. It works.

"Since my hysterectomy when my ovaries were removed, I have lost my interest in sex. This doesn't suit me, or my husband either. Are there any solutions?"

A tiny dose of testosterone taken alone or with the estrogen can help rekindle sexual feelings, increase energy levels, and overcome vaginal atrophy at the same time. A shortage of androgens, easily detected by a simple blood test, not only leads to possible loss of libido and sensory responses but also can lower the rate and quality of orgasm and, in some women, induces depression and lethargy, especially among women who have had surgical menopause. In fact, studies at McGill University in Montreal have shown that small doses of testosterone given to postmenopausal women dramatically increases their sexual desire.

"How quickly does this treatment work?"

According to Gloria A. Bachmann, M.D., a specialist in the medical aspects of human sexuality, daily doses should produce an increase in libido within only three to five days. Androgens are not taken just prior to intercourse but intermittently for several days at a time, usually in tablet form, alone, or combined with estrogen. They can also be taken by injection or by slow-release subcutaneous pellets.

"Are there any masculinizing effects from taking male hormones? I wouldn't want to grow a mustache or start talking in a deep voice."

The only adverse side effect noted so far is the growth of hair on the chin and upper lip when testosterone is taken in large doses over long periods. But with low-dose treatment this is not likely to happen to you. Even if it does, the problem is reversible when the dose is lowered even more. Voice deepening is rare and it, too, is reversible by cutting the dose.

"Is it possible that the medication I take for high blood pressure is having an effect on my sex drive? I've read that it can cause problems in men, but how about women?"

Check that out with your doctor, who can switch you to another drug for hypertension or lower your dose. Many blood pressure medications including diuretics can dampen libido. So can some common antianxiety drugs such as Valium and Xanax, antidepressants like Elavil, and antiulcer medications such as Tagamet and Zantac. These medications can interfere with sexual function in several ways: you may lose interest in sex, produce less vaginal lubrication, or have difficulty reaching orgasm.

"Can regular exercise increase libido?"

Yes, although indirectly. Several large studies of men and women have found that regular exercise enhances libido. If that's true, it's probably because it tones the body, boosts energy, relieves stress, and acts as an antidepressant.

PREVENTIONS AND REMEDIES

Although hormone replacement therapy is the ultimate answer to uncomfortable sex, let's talk first about other ways to prevent sexual suicide.

Use a Lubricant If your only apparent problem now is vaginal dryness, use a lubricant to prevent the uncomfortable friction of a penis against your fragile vaginal lining. Dab a goodly amount on the penis or the vaginal opening (or both) just prior to intercourse. Never use a lubricant that is not designed for this specific purpose, especially oil-based products such as petroleum jelly, cocoa butter, or baby oil. Not only will they cake and dry, making the situation much worse by blocking whatever natural secretions you are still producing, but they can also destroy latex condoms (only latex condoms should be used for protection against sexually transmitted diseases), creating little holes for viruses and sperm to pass through. And don't use vaginal moisturizers as lubricants, either. They don't do a good lubricating job and, besides, they are acidic and could cause your partner some discomfort.

Use *only* water-soluble, oil-free, nonstaining, odorless "personal lubricants" made specifically for this purpose, such as K-Y Jelly, Astroglide, Lubrin, Surgilube, Maxilube, Transi-Lube, and Ortho Personal Lubricant. By the way, water-soluble lubricants do not interfere with the effectiveness of spermicides.

> Vitamin E oil is the only exception to the above rule because it doesn't dry or cake and may even help relieve irritation. Forget almond or coconut oil, although some women swear by them, maybe because they taste good. Their high sugar content encourages fungal infections.

If you feel discomfort not only during penetration but also during active intercourse, try a lubricating suppository such as Lubrin vaginal lubricating inserts or Lubafax, in addition to the lubricant gel, inserting it into the vagina where it will quickly dissolve. Start with the half-size suppositories, which may be enough, then graduate to the full size if you find you need them.

Use a Vaginal Moisturizer Nonhormonal vaginal moisturizers—such as Replens, Moist Again, and Gyne-Moistrin—hydrate the cells of the vaginal lining, allowing them to build up a continually moist protective layer. An added advantage is that they have a very low pH, which means they are acidic and can therefore help maintain a healthy vaginal environment discouraging to unfriendly infection-causing bacteria that migrate over from the urinary tract or the rectum.

Although estrogen replacement does a far superior job of restoring your vagina to its former functional self because it actually regenerates the protective layer of cornified cells, thereby treating the underlying cause of the problem, the moisturizers significantly increase moisture and elasticity in the majority of women who use them.

Inserted into the vagina with a disposable applicator about three times a week, preferably in the morning, a moisturizer can relieve dryness for days at a time. Helpful for premenopausal women whose vaginas have only just begun to show the results of an estrogen deficiency, they work best if you start using them as soon as dryness begins to be a problem. They are also a useful alternative to HRT for those past menopause who can't or don't wish to take hormones.

Beware of Antihistamines and Other Drugs

Antihistamines and certain decongestants, designed to dry the mucus membranes of your nasal passages, will also dry out your vagina, adding to your difficulties. So use them sparingly. Other drugs, including cardiovascular medications, antidepressants, atropine drugs, and diuretics may do the same.

Speaking of drugs, too much alcohol may relax your inhibitions but it also tends to decrease sexual arousal and discourage orgasm.

Maintain an Active Sex Life Continued sexual intercourse can help maintain your sexual responsiveness and keep your vagina more supple, elastic, and lubricated, lessening the likelihood that sex will become painful. Regular sexual activity (including masturbation, oral sex, manual stimulation, and the use of mechanical aids) increases the blood flow to your sexual organs, stimulates the glands that secrete lubrication, and retards the atrophic changes, including pH alkalinity and dryness. In other words, use it or lose it.

Most sexual problems are not hormonal, however, but are due to an "antierotic" atmosphere—poor communications between sex partners concerning their needs and desires, poor personal hygiene, perfunctory foreplay, or too little romance. Sometimes sex counseling or therapy, perhaps in addition to hormones, is the answer.

Take a Sitz Bath This will help to relieve acute irritation, itching, or burning.

Practice the Kegel Exercises To strengthen your pelvic muscles and improve vaginal tone, exercise this area of your body as many times a day as you think of it (see page 320). Repeatedly squeeze and relax the muscles you would contract to stop urination, holding for up to ten seconds, working up to at least twenty-five times each session. Or do it this way: whenever you urinate, intermittently start and stop the flow, holding it back for ten seconds each time.

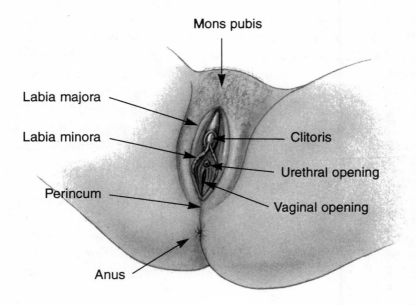

Take the Pill If you are still having menstrual periods, you still need pregnancy protection. The low-dose combination birth-control pills can not only serve as protection but, because they contain estrogen, also help keep your vagina in good condition. What's more, they will keep erratic periods under control, regulating them so they are predictable, and suppress early perimenopausal symptoms at the same time (see Chapters 2 and 9).

Use Vaginal Estrogen Cream If the moisturizers don't restore your vaginal lining enough to make sexual intercourse comfortable once more, and you are not a prime candidate for osteoporosis or heart disease (if you are, you need oral or transdermal estrogen), then it makes good sense to ask your doctor for a prescription for vaginal estrogen cream. The cream *is* a form of estrogen replacement, but very little of the hormone is absorbed into the bloodstream after you have used it long enough to rejuvenate your vagina. How much and how often you use the cream depends on your needs. Some women don't absorb it as well as others and require higher doses. Except in unusual cases, it's best to begin with a relatively high dose—perhaps 2 grams three times a week for two weeks—and then cut back to 1 gram, a low dose, twice a week. As the damage is repaired and the vagina is restored to good condition, you will absorb less and less of the hormone into your bloodstream. You can maintain your own schedule with vaginal cream, starting and stopping it as necessary, but, unless you start using another form of HRT, you will always have to go back to it on a fairly regular schedule. Sometimes, even with HRT by pill or patch, you will need vaginal cream too, if only occasionally.

If you use estrogen cream, remember that *some* of the hormone is absorbed, just like estrogen taken any other way. So if you still possess a uterus, you must visit your gynecologist regularly to be sure you are not developing hyperplasia, an excessively thick uterine lining that, when neglected, can lead to cancer. If you are found to have hyperplasia, you must take progesterone too, at least periodically.

Most important, report any bleeding that occurs while you are on estrogen cream. Bleeding may mean hyperplasia, which means you must take progesterone *now*. Vaginal bleeding that's not according to plan must *always* be thoroughly investigated.

Watch for the new vaginal ring from Sweden, now being evaluated by the Food and Drug Administration, and ask your doctor about using it. Called Estring, the ring is placed in the vagina, much like a diaphragm, where it slowly releases minute amounts of estradiol—a form of estrogen—which restores the vaginal lining and its ability to lubricate itself, but is not absorbed into the bloodstream to affect other parts of the body.

Take Estrogen Replacement Although all of the above will certainly help you preserve your sex life, estrogen replacement by pill or patch is the ultimate answer. Lubricants, moisturizers, and other measures do not supply this key ingredient that restores the vagina's original structure, its sensitivity, and its own ability to provide lubrication when sexually stimulated. So if you are having a serious problem in bed and if there is no medical reason why you can't take estrogen, we suggest you move right along to HRT after menopause.

Hormone replacement will end your sexual difficulties very quickly. You'll start seeing results in only a couple of weeks when blood flow to the pelvic area increases, the vaginal lining begins to toughen up, lubrication improves, touch perception improves, and the itchiness and soreness are alleviated. And in a month or two (longer if you have really let yourself go), you will probably be as good as new. If you still have vaginal symptoms, ask your gynecologist about taking a higher dose of estrogen and/or using vaginal cream in addition to your pill or patch.

Can Vitamins Help?

It's scientifically uncertain whether vitamin supplements can help boost sexual desire, but vitamin E has been credited with good results and so have the B vitamins. In any case, a healthy diet that consistently contains all of the essential nutrients certainly won't hurt.

"I've been using vaginal douches for years because they make me feel cleaner. But I was told they can encourage dryness. Is this true?"

Yes. Douching can strip away natural moisture and cause dryness. Besides, you don't need it. The only douche that can possibly do you any good for any reason whatsoever is a simple vinegar-and-water preparation that makes your vagina more acidic and therefore more resistant to infections.

"Are you ever beyond repair? I haven't been able to have sex for years because it became excruciatingly painful. Now I am thinking of marrying again."

No matter how long your vagina has been out of circulation (except in the most extreme cases), it can be made functional again. Sometimes, however, if you have been celibate for a very long time, you may need special help: perhaps higher than usual doses of estrogen at first in addition to regular applications of vaginal estrogen cream. This is something you will have to work out with your doctor, so give yourself time for repairs before having sex again.

Occasionally, of course, women let themselves go for so long that they suffer from really severe vaginal atrophy. In that case, a vaginal dilator, a device that gradually stretches the vagina, may be necessary for a while along with hormone replacement to help widen the contracted passageway.

"If I use vaginal estrogen cream, can it affect my boyfriend?"

Making love with estrogen cream in your vagina probably won't affect him one way or the other, but it is a waste of the medication. Use it after intercourse, or in the morning, or on a night when you are not anticipating sex.

"I invariably develop a urinary infection after I have sex. Can I do anything to prevent this?"

Yes. See Chapter 15.

"My vulva tends to get very dry and itchy and sometimes even sore. What should I put on it?"

Treat it just as you would dry skin anywhere else on your body, using an unscented lubricating skin cream. Just be careful not to get the cream in your vagina, where it may be irritating. Or try a thin film of vitamin E oil once or twice a day.

"Is it normal to take much longer to become aroused as you get older?"

Definitely, although it happens for some women and not for others.

"I seem to have one vaginal infection after another lately, and I always have burning, irritation, and sometimes bleeding when I have intercourse. What can I do to put a stop to this pattern?"

Check out the suggestions above (and see Chapter 11). Restoring your vagina with HRT or, to a lesser degree with a vaginal moisturizer, will do wonders, while using a lubricant and following the other advice will help, too. But first make sure you are not passing an infection back and forth between you and your partner, in which case you should both be treated simultaneously with antibiotics.

Vaginitis, a catchall term for various viral, bacterial, or yeast infections, can make you miserable all the time but especially during intercourse. If you treat it as soon as the symptoms start, you will have a better chance of clearing it up fast. Chronic cases can be very stubborn. Don't assume it will go away on its own. Go to your doctor to have the infection identified and a medication prescribed, at least the first time around. Avoid medicated douches, feminine hygiene sprays, deodorant tampons, and perfumed soaps—all of which can be irritating and drying. Never use tampons when your vagina is burning or bleeding. Also, if you have a tendency to get vaginitis, stay out of whirlpools and hot tubs, even your own. See Chapter 11 for more on vaginitis.

"I have just found out I have diabetes. I've read that women with diabetes have sexual problems. Is this true?"

Women with insulin-dependent diabetes frequently do face special sexual difficulties. High blood sugar, for example, may result in decreased libido and arousal as well as a reduction in vaginal lubrication and tends to encourage vaginal infections, especially yeast, which thrives on the glucose in vaginal secretions. As you get older, the problems are compounded by your diminishing estrogen supply. So what can you do about all these possibilities? Keep your blood sugar under very tight control with regular self-monitoring, diet, and exercise, as well as your insulin or oral medications.

It's also an excellent idea to take high-dose B complex vitamins, perhaps a B-100 tablet every day, for peripheral neuropathy. It can help repair the peripheral nerves that affect sexual arousal.

"If I am already taking oral estrogen, can I still use a vaginal moisturizer?"

Yes, if you think you need one. You will not be adding more estrogen because the moisturizers do not contain hormones. But if you take estrogen supplements and still have an uncomfortably dry vagina, talk it over with your doctor. Perhaps your estrogen dose is too low. The dose must be individualized because some women require more estrogen than others to produce the same results. Or perhaps it would be a good idea to use vaginal estrogen cream topically for a while—in addition to the estrogen pills—at least until your vagina is in better shape.

"I have nowhere near as much pleasure from sex since my hysterectomy. Why not?"

Were your ovaries removed too? If so, that's the reason and the only good answer is hormone replacement therapy, perhaps including androgens. Some women also report that they get extra pleasure from contractions of the uterus during sex and, if you were among them, you may miss it now.

SEX AFTER BREAST CANCER

Breast cancer, especially if it results in mastectomy, obviously has tremendous emotional consequences and effects on feelings about sexuality. And it also has major effects on your physical ability to have and enjoy sex because of the side effects of the treatment you may be given to prevent a recurrence.

Chemotherapy usually destroys ovarian function, causing premature menopause and a loss of both estrogen and testosterone, affecting both the physical ability to have comfortable sex and the enjoyment of sexual activity. The sudden menopause, with its severe hot flashes, almost immediate vaginal dryness, and other symptoms, certainly can dampen sexual pleasure by turning sex into an abrasive business. At the same time, the loss of hormones suppresses your libido.

Tamoxifen, an antiestrogenic drug commonly used in breast-cancer patients today as an alternative to chemotherapy, is less toxic than chemotherapy and doesn't have such a deleterious effect on sexuality. Although it blocks the body's use of estrogen, resulting in especially powerful hot flashes and vaginal dryness, it also acts as a weak estrogen in some ways so that helps strengthen bones and protect the heart, and the vaginal problems women experience with its use are usually nowhere near as severe as with chemotherapy.

Some women taking tamoxifen report a decline in libido and orgastic response, which may be a sign of androgen deficiency resulting from the use of the drug. But, says Dr. Kaplan, of the New York Hospital-Cornell Medical Center, "in contrast to chemotherapy, which can leave permanent damage, the adverse effects of TAM on libido and on orgasm are entirely reversible upon cessation of medication and can, in some cases, be improved by lowering the daily dose."

"Is there anything to be done to relieve drenching hot flashes that occur at least every hour day and night if you have had breast cancer and estrogen is forbidden?"

Ask your doctor about taking Megace, the only kind of progesterone that has been approved by the FDA for women who have had breast cancer. It often provides some relief for hot flashes and the other typical symptoms of estrogen deprivation. Megace, in fact, is sometimes used as treatment after breast cancer because it can stop the growth of abnormal cells.

Also try taking vitamin E and heeding the other suggestions in Chapter 3.

"I have had breast cancer so my doctor says I can never take estrogen. But I absolutely cannot have sex without pain anymore. What do you suggest I do?"

You may have little choice but to tough it out. If you have had estrogen-dependent breast cancer, the general opinion is that you cannot take HRT except perhaps for vaginal estrogen cream *if* your oncologist agrees.

In our own practice, however, we have found that only 1 gram of vaginal cream inserted into the vagina once a week helps to make the vagina much more functional. This is a very tiny dose compared to the standard recommendation of 4 grams four times a week, and because it is so small, it is unlikely to be absorbed into the bloodstream where it might accelerate the growth of any remaining cancer cells. Unlikely or not, your blood estrogen levels should be checked regularly while you are on this regime.

But there are other measures that may be quite effective, especially if you start them very early. Try twice-daily applications of vaginal moisturizer such as Replens, Gyne-Moistrin, or Moist Again, both during and following chemotherapy or tamoxifen treatment. Dr. Kaplan also suggests intercourse, with lubricants, on a regular basis and/or the use of vaginal dilators to keep the passageway open if intercourse occurs less than once a week.

Many cancer specialists see no reason to prohibit testosterone treatment for women with breast cancer if they have a loss of libido because of an androgen deficiency, although there is still some controversy about this. Substitutes for testosterone replacement, not nearly as effective, include the drugs Wellbutrin and Eldepryl. In addition, Megace, which is progesterone, sometimes helps to increase sexual desire.

Because it is extremely difficult to differentiate between psychogenic sexual difficulties that result from having had breast cancer and the effect of physical deficits that can be produced by cancer treatments, we suggest in-depth discussions with your oncologist, gynecologist, and perhaps a psychotherapist.

Another remedy that may prove to be a boon to women who have had breast cancer and therefore can't take HRT in its usual forms may be approved for breast-cancer patients in this country before long. This is Estring, a vaginal estrogen ring, currently available in Sweden. Inserted in the vagina against the cervix and changed every twelve weeks, it releases a very tiny amount (5 micrograms) of estrogen a day—just enough to restore the vaginal tissues but not enough to be absorbed into the bloodstream. Meanwhile it increases vaginal lubrication and elasticity.

"Do all chemotherapy treatments result in a permanent menopause?"

No, although the older you are, the more likely it is that they will. Some relatively gentle drugs cause only a temporary ovarian shutdown, allowing you to get your periods back after the treatment ends.

"Is it an absolute rule that breast-cancer patients can't take hormone replacement therapy?"

Many specialists are now rethinking the ban on estrogen for cancer survivors, and a current study is investigating the risks of HRT for women with breast cancer. Meanwhile, because all the results aren't in yet, you are the one who must make the final decision.

Chapter 8

SEXUALLY TRANSMITTED DISEASES: A CONCERN AT ANY AGE

IT'S NEVER TOO LATE to get a sexually transmitted disease. In fact, it's even easier to get one now that your vagina is becoming dryer, more fragile, and less acidic. The truth is, the dryer and more easily abraded it gets as time goes by, the greater your risk of catching a disease you definitely don't want. Even if you take hormone replacement therapy after menopause, your vagina will never be as sturdy as a 30-year-old's. So don't think, just because you are 40, 50, or even 80, that you are safe unless you are celibate. And don't think either that you can't catch a sexually transmitted disease (STD) from an older man. It requires only one unprotected sexual encounter with an infected person, whatever age, to come away with a big problem.

Although the issues of STDs have always been of primary interest to younger women who usually have more sexual partners, they have begun to apply more and more to women in their middle years. Today many older women are changing partners, acquiring new ones, or having multiple encounters, thereby putting themselves at risk. They represent a small but growing segment of the AIDS epidemic as well. So even if your doctor may not consider you a likely candidate for STDs or may refuse a request to be screened, insist on it unless you are *absolutely* certain you are in a mutually monogamous long-term relationship.

Older Americans are in a state of denial about their risk of getting one of the millions of cases of STDs reported every year. Those over 50 are six times less likely to use condoms and five times less likely to get tested for AIDS than people in their twenties with similar risk factors, although they have the highest rate of heterosexual transmission, according to epidemiologists at the University of California at San Francisco.

Your risk of getting an STD, whatever your age, is directly related to how many sexual partners you have had *and* how many sexual partners your partners have had. STDs are at epidemic levels today, and an estimated one in five Americans has contracted one. They are, in fact, the third most common infections in the United States, right after colds and the flu. They are most prevalent among 15- to 37-year-olds, as you would expect, but nobody's immune. Although AIDS is the most lethal and the most publicized, there are several others that may not kill you but can certainly affect the quality of your life.

WHAT ARE STDS?

Sexually transmitted diseases are infections primarily passed along through vaginal or anal intercourse and frequently through oral sex as well. Flourishing in dark, moist, warm places inside the body, they include bacterial infections like gonorrhea or chlamydia that are treatable with antibiotics, and viral diseases like herpes that can be controlled but never cured. They may not always cause obvious symptoms and rarely go away on their own. All of them have potentially serious consequences if they are not treated.

STDs affect women disproportionately because women tend to show fewer symptoms than men, experience more complications, and often go untreated until permanent damage is done. Perhaps, even more important, women are much more likely to get an STD from men than the other way around.

How Not to Get an STD

There are only two ways to protect yourself against STDs if you are sexually active:

- Limit your partners to *one* person who you are *absolutely certain* does not have an STD.
- Use a latex condom (not one made of a natural membrane because viruses can sneak through its pores) in combination with a cream or jelly containing the spermicide nonoxynol 9, with all sexual activity until a mutually monogamous relationship has been in effect for *at least* three months. Then continue using the condom until both of you have been tested for HIV antibody. Almost everyone who is infected is found to have positive antibodies when tested within three months of contracting the disease. Although a condom does not guarantee protection from STDs, it is the most effective available barrier against them.
- Avoid frequent douching, which is associated with an increased risk of pelvic inflammatory disease (PID), which in turn is caused by STDs.
- Stop smoking. It can impair the immune system.

How to Use a Condom Correctly *

- Always use a good-quality latex (rubber) condom, not natural membrane (lambskin) or novelty items. Use it in combination with the spermicide nonoxynol 9 to protect you from disease and pregnancy.
- Store condoms in a cool dry place, not in your wallet or glove compartment. Air, heat, and light weaken the latex.
- Be careful not to rip the condom with teeth or nails when opening the wrapper. Never reuse a condom. Use a new one for each new act of intercourse, whether vaginal, anal, or oral.
- Apply the condom to an erect penis *before* there is any contact between penis and vagina.
- If extra lubrication is needed, use a water-soluble cream or gel made specifically for this purpose. Do *not* use an oil-based lubricant such as petroleum jelly, cocoa butter, shortening, body lotion, or oil, which can destroy the rubber.
- Do not use condoms after their expiration date stamped on the wrapper. Never use condoms that are damaged, discolored, brittle, or sticky.

*Source: Centers for Disease Control.

"Do I have to use a condom even though I have had a tubal ligation?"

Just because you have been sterilized and can't get pregnant, it doesn't mean you can't get a sexually transmitted disease. The same is true for a man who has had a vasectomy. Sterilization protects you from pregnancy but does not help you avoid diseases. Neither does any other form of contraception except for condoms in combination with spermicide.

"I have had a hysterectomy. Does that provide any protection?"

No. Infections are transmitted through the mucous membranes and blood access, not through the uterus. Although your fallopian tubes (if they were removed) are no longer at risk for pelvic inflammatory disease (PID), you can still get vaginal and blood-borne infections.

"Are women who use oral contraceptives more likely to get an STD?"

The pill does not make you more vulnerable to STDs, and it even provides some protection against PID. However, if women who use oral contraceptives have many sexual partners and/or do not use condoms regularly, their risk increases accordingly.

"Does hormone replacement therapy make you more or less susceptible to these diseases?"

Nobody knows for sure yet, but it doesn't matter very much because any woman who has sexual contact with an infected partner is at risk for infection, no matter what her hormonal status.

THE COMMON STDs

GONORRHEA AND CHLAMYDIA

Chlamydia is currently the most common bacterial STD in the United States, and one of the most potentially damaging. Gonorrhea and chlamydia often travel together. Twenty-five to 50 percent of women with gonorrhea (at its highest level in almost half a century) will also test positive for chlamydia. And, in fact, patients who are diagnosed for gonorrhea should automatically be treated for its companion disease, which is harder to detect.

Untreated, gonorrhea and chlamydia can infect the fallopian tubes and ovaries, producing pelvic inflammatory disease (PID) that, in turn, causes infertility, ectopic pregnancies, and chronic pain.

Symptoms: Both of these STDs are often "silent," causing no symptoms at all, but sometimes they cause pain or burning on urination, an inflamed cervix, pain during intercourse and spotting after it, and a vaginal discharge. Up to three-quarters of cases in women have no symptoms, at least for long periods of time. When symptoms do occur, however, they usually make an appearance within a week to three weeks after the initial exposure.

In men, chlamydia may produce only mild symptoms, perhaps itching inside the urethra or a stinging sensation, a discharge, or uncomfortable urination. But men, too, may have no symptoms at all and meanwhile they continue to transmit the disease to every woman they sleep with. Gonorrhea usually results in an infectious discharge that may prompt its male victims to seek medical attention.

Treatment: Chlamydia and gonorrhea can be readily cured *if* your sexual partner(s) are also treated, whether they have symptoms or not. The usual treatment is seven to ten days of doxycycline (an antibiotic of the tetracycline family) or erythromycin.

What to do now: Ask your doctor for a gonorrhea-chlamydia test, especially if you have a new partner or more than one partner. A new laboratory test gives results in four hours.

PID (PELVIC INFLAMMATORY DISEASE)

This is a catchall term for a variety of painful infections of the upper reproductive organs: the uterus, the ovaries, the fallopian tubes, and sometimes the entire pelvic area. It is the result of infection by some of the sexually transmitted diseases (primarily gonorrhea and chlamydia) and sometimes by combinations of common vaginal bacteria. Unless promptly treated, it can have serious long-term complications, including infertility, ectopic pregnancy, and chronic pain.

Symptoms: The symptoms of PID often start during or shortly after a menstrual period and include severe lower abdominal and pelvic pain, perhaps accompanied by fever, vaginal discharge, and nausea. If in doubt about the diagnosis, your doctor may recommend a laparoscopy so that the uterus, tubes, and ovaries may be directly viewed with a fiberoptic scope.

Treatment: Antibiotics, sometimes oral, but frequently intravenous, which requires hospitalization.

What to do now: Make sure you are properly treated for the underlying infection—usually gonorrhea or chlamydia, which may not themselves produce any noticeable symptoms. Both are curable.

HUMAN PAPILLOMA VIRUS (HPV)

Also called condyloma, this virus causes genital warts in some of its victims and is the prime suspect in nearly all cervical cancer (see Chapter 13). It is the most common viral STD in the United States, with 24 to 40 million cases and over a million new ones diagnosed each year. Not always symptomatic, it can remain latent for years. It is highly contagious, giving you a 50 percent chance of getting it with just one sexual encounter. To date, there is no cure for HPV. It takes up permanent residence in your body, so once you've got it, you've got it for life, although it may vanish and then reappear in fresh outbreaks weeks or months later.

Symptoms: Genital warts (in about 10 percent of the cases) and dysplasia. The tiny warts, itchy perhaps but usually painless, may appear one to three months after exposure, although you may be asymptomatic for longer. Singly or in clusters, they may appear externally on the vulva or peritoneum or internally in the vagina, anus, or cervix, where your gynecologist may be the first to notice them. Or perhaps they become sore or start to bleed, especially after intercourse. Their appearance varies, but they usually look like small cauliflowerlike pinkish skin tags.

A Pap test will detect the dysplasia—abnormalities in the cervical tissue—that accompanies the human papilloma virus. Left untreated, it can possibly develop into cancer over time.

Treatment: The warts can be destroyed by freezing with liquid nitrogen, applications of trichloracetic acid, injections of interferon, laser treatment, or electrosurgery. Dysplasia must be removed.

What to do now: Be sure to have a Pap test at least once a year, more often if you have tested positive for HPV or have signs of dysplasia. Always use condoms.

For helpful information about STDs:

The American Social Health Association
P.O. Box 13827
Research Triangle Park, NC 27709
919-361-8400
or call the
National STD Hotline
800-227-8922

GENITAL HERPES

This condition is caused by the herpes simplex virus, transmitted by skin-to-skin contact with an infected partner. While some people have no symptoms at all or merely a genital tingling, it can produce exquisitely painful sores that look like blisters.

Recurrent and currently incurable, herpes has reached epidemic proportions as every year more Americans join the ranks of the 40 million who are already infected. After the initial exposure, the virus causes its first attack within a few days to a week. This virus, like HPV, never leaves you, although it goes into inactive, or latent, phases and then emerges again to cause an active infection that may be triggered by stress, menstruation, or illness. The first attack is usually the worst, with subsequent outbreaks gradually becoming less severe, less frequent, and less prolonged.

Remember that it is possible to contract genital herpes from contact with a cold sore (also caused by the herpes simplex virus) during oral sex.

Symptoms: Although some herpes victims have no symptoms and others only minor ones, most develop painful sores on and around the genitals. These are often accompanied, at least in the first attack, by uncomfortable urination, swollen lymph nodes in the groin, and flulike symptoms such as fever, aches, fatigue, and headache. The sores may signal their imminent arrival by itching or tingling or stabbing pains. The blisters form scabs that fall off within two to three weeks.

Treatment: After a tissue culture confirms the diagnosis of genital herpes, the symptoms can be greatly alleviated and the outbreaks shortened by Zovirax (acyclovir) started as soon as symptoms appear and taken five times a day for five to ten days. For women who have many recurrences a year, Zovirax taken two to five times a day may keep the virus under control. This drug may soon be available without a prescription and new drugs, variations of acyclovir, are awaiting FDA approval.

Although acyclovir is currently the only treatment for genital herpes, an experimental vaccine seems to boost the body's immune response to the disease and reduce by a third the number of outbreaks in people with previous recurrences.

The vaccine may turn out to be another way to keep the virus under control.

What to do now: Don't have sex when you feel tingling or have active sores. Always use condoms plus a spermicide containing nonoxynol 9 to avoid spreading the infection. You must practice this safe sex at all times, whether or not you have sores at the moment or you are taking the medication, because at least 5 percent of women can pass the virus along even when it is in a latent phase. During an outbreak, don't touch the affected area because the virus can be transmitted by contaminated fingers.

AIDS (AUTOIMMUNE DEFICIENCY SYNDROME)

You are at risk for AIDS as well as other STDs if you have intercourse with a man whose sperm carries the virus. So be assertive and always insist that an untested partner use condoms (plus spermicide), which aside from celibacy, remains the most effective method of protection against HIV (human immunodeficiency virus). An estimated 100,000 American women are currently infected with HIV, 25 percent of them over the age of 40.

FAST FACTS ABOUT AIDS

- Women are three to five times more likely to contract the AIDS virus from an infected partner than men are to get it from women. Sexual intercourse is now the most common way for women to contract the disease.
- Women die 20 percent sooner than men after their first symptoms.
- Currently, women make up 11 percent of AIDS cases.
- Many STDs, including HIV, occur concurrently. So

you should be tested for HIV whenever you are tested for any of the others.
• Possible warning signals include symptoms of other STDs, persistent swollen lymph nodes, frequent fevers and sweats, constantly recurring yeast infections, weight loss.

Not me? Never assume, because you are a respectable, midlife, middle-class woman, that you can't possibly get AIDS. If you have had more than one sexual partner in the past year and have not used a condom with every encounter, have yourself tested, whether or not your doctor considers you a likely candidate.

For information and referrals, call:

The National AIDS Hotline
800-227-8922

Chapter 9
===

BIRTH CONTROL:
WHAT'S YOUR OPTION NOW?

IF YOU WOULD BE LESS THAN DELIGHTED by an unplanned pregnancy at this time in your life, be sure to use effective contraception every time you have intercourse until you are certifiably menopausal. If you don't, you may have to make some big decisions that weren't on your agenda. Although it is true that you probably aren't as fertile as you once were—fertility declines with every passing year, leaving only about half of women still fertile at age 41 and one in ten at age 45—it certainly is possible to get pregnant in your forties, sometimes (though rarely) even in your fifties. In fact, the percentage of women over 40 having elective abortions is second only to teenagers.

You can't count on being absolutely infertile until menopause; even then, it's advisable to use contraception for at least six months after your last menstrual period, just in case your ovaries decide to make one last try at turning out an egg. What confuses many women is perimenopause—the time when your body is preparing to end its reproductive days, when your periods and ovulation tend to be erratic and strange. If you follow the typical perimenopausal pattern, you'll skip periods here and there. Or the periods will stop for a while and then start up again, maybe vanishing for several months before returning for several more. Meanwhile, you may think you can't get pregnant—but you can. Every now and then your ovaries may turn out a viable egg, an egg that may manage to meet up with an energetic sperm and become fertilized. Now is the time to decide whether or not you want to take that chance.

Now is also an excellent time to take a good look at your contraception method and decide whether the one you've been using still suits your needs. Many changes in birth control have occurred in the last few years, and your life may well have changed, too. The kind of contraception you chose at 25 or 30 may not be what you need today.

WHAT YOUR CHOICES ARE *NOW*

The contraception that's right for you depends on your lifestyle. If you are in a mutually monogamous relationship, the full range of options is open whatever your age because you don't have to be concerned about acquiring a sexually transmitted disease, although the new combination oral contraceptives offer special advantages that can ease you through perimenopause. If you have multiple or serial partners, or you're not sure what your future holds, then your choice narrows down to one: condoms (with spermicide for added protection), *regardless* of whether you are already using another, more permanent method.

Two-thirds of women over 40 have ended their chances of reproduction with tubal ligations or their partners' vasectomies. Sterilization is the most effective method of all and, besides, may possibly lower the risk of ovarian cancer. Its ability to prevent pregnancy is closely matched by Norplant, followed by the hormonal oral contraceptives and the IUD (intrauterine device), all of which have the advantage of allowing sexual spontaneity, although they have higher risks of pregnancy and a few side effects. The barrier and spermicide methods have fewer side effects but require motivation, discipline, and effort. Besides, some women find them too bothersome or messy. Unfortunately, the perfect method of contraception has yet to come along, so you just have to pick the one that works best for you.

Remember that you have *no* choice when you are having intercourse with a person you don't know well, isn't your permanent monogamous partner, and may not be 100 percent reliable when he says he never sleeps with anyone else. Even then, he may be carrying a disease from earlier relationships and doesn't know it. Use a condom. Period. Use it *whether or not* you are already using another method of contraception. Never take a chance, not even once.

Just in case you think it is ever worth taking a chance, consider these facts: AIDS will kill you. Viral STDs, such as human papilloma and herpes, while they are not lethal, can never be cured. Other STDs may not last a lifetime, but they can cause serious problems that do.

THE PILL: A GOOD CHOICE IN PERIMENOPAUSE

Until very recently, only 5 percent of women over 35 and 3 percent over 40 were using oral contraceptives. But now "the pill" has become the birth-control method of choice for many older women, an estimated half a million of them between the ages of 45 and 50. That's because this method, more than 30 years old and investigated more than any other medication in the world, has been vastly improved since the days of flower power.

The newest very-low-dose combination oral contraceptives

contain only about a fifth the estrogen and less than half the progesterone of the earlier versions, and have been declared safe by the FDA for healthy women right up to the age of 50 or menopause, whichever comes first. Many early concerns about its links to cardiovascular problems were based on preparations with much higher doses of estrogen than are used today and no longer apply. (Also available are oral contraceptives with no estrogen. Called progestin-only or mini-pills, they are for women who can't take estrogen; see page 198.)

A boon to perimenopausal women who are always wondering whether a skipped period means pregnancy or menopause, oral contraceptives not only do an excellent job of preventing pregnancy (with less than 1 percent failure rate when used properly) but they also give you estrogen and progesterone in a safe, low dose that regulates erratic periods and stops hot flashes. At the same time, they enhance bone density and probably protect you against heart attacks.

Even better, oral contraceptives taken long term have been found to decrease the risk of ovarian and endometrial cancer by more than 50 percent, with the protection lasting for at least fifteen years after you quit. In fact, the risk reduction for ovarian cancer is so impressive that the pill is often prescribed for women with family histories of this disease. Women taking the pill also have fewer ovarian cysts and benign breast tumors.

Questions about the connection between the new pill and the risk of breast cancer have not been definitively answered, but the evidence to date suggests it doesn't affect the risk appreciably one way or the other.

Current thinking is that the low-dose pill—a combination of estrogen and protesterone—can be safely used (if you are a nonsmoker) at least until the age of 50. Then if you are menopausal, you can move right on to hormone replacement therapy (HRT) without skipping a beat. HRT is preferred at this time because, unlike the pill, it does not compete with your own hormone production but instead adds to it.

Who Should *Not* Use the Pill

Oral contraceptives, even very-low-dose, have their limitations. You are advised to choose another form of contraception if you:

- Are a smoker
- Have a history of angina, heart attack, or stroke, or are at high risk for same
- Have a history of phlebitis, thrombophlebitis, or other kinds of circulatory or clotting abnormalities
- Suffer from migraines or depression that are exacerbated by the hormones in the pill
- Have known or suspected breast, endometrial, or cervical cancer, or a liver tumor

"Why can't you use it if you are a smoker?"

A smoker has two pill-related problems. First, smoking interferes with the absorption of the hormones in the pill, so it's possible to get an insufficient dose and end up pregnant. Second, all of smoking's bad effects are accentuated by the pill, including clotting problems that could lead to stroke or heart attack.

"Can you take the pill if you have diabetes?"

Yes, if you use the newest pills, which contain so little estrogen and progestin that they have little if any effect on metabolism.

"What's different about the new birth-control pills?"

The early oral contraceptives, besides having many annoying side effects, could elevate blood pressure, damage the liver, and in susceptible women, cause blood clots, coronary artery damage, and stroke. The current low-dose pills with only 20 percent of the estrogen in the originals are considered safe for healthy women over 40 who do not smoke and have no other risk factors.

"How does the combination pill work?"

In several ways. First, it suppresses the production of LH (luteinizing hormone) and prevents ovulation. It renders the uterine lining unreceptive to an egg even if it does manage to ovulate. And it makes the cervical mucus hostile to sperm. It is taken for three weeks on, one week off, to allow time for a menstrual period.

"How will you know if you've had menopause when you are taking the pill?"

You probably won't, unless you stop taking it for a week or two and have your FSH level measured. If that level is over 40 mIU/ml (microinternational units per milliliter), your ovaries have stopped working and, if you like, you can switch directly to hormone replacement therapy. If you do it this way, you'll never have menopausal symptoms—or bone loss either, for that matter. You could even stay on the pills after menopause, using them as replacement, although it may supply more hormones than you need. HRT, which contains even lower amounts, is preferred for that reason.

"What are the side effects of taking oral contraceptives? I took them once and gained a lot of weight."

Weight gain (almost always less than five pounds) is one of the possible side effects and so is breakthrough bleeding or spotting. The new pills, unlike the old, don't usually cause headaches, breast tenderness, acne, nausea, moodiness, or depression. But if they do, these side effects will probably fade after the first few cycles. If they continue, experiment with different brands to try to find one that agrees with you before you give up.

"How come some women get pregnant even though they're on the pill?"

The usual reason for getting pregnant on birth-control pills is forgetting to take them or stopping and starting them according to the status of your sex life. With the old formula you could probably get away with skipping a day or two, but today you can't count on that. To be on the safe side if you miss a day with low-dose pills, use condoms, a diaphragm, or at least a spermicide along with the pills for the rest of that *entire* cycle.

As we've mentioned, smoking in combination with the pill may lower the absorption of the hormones and provide another way of becoming pregnant when you thought you were absolutely safe.

"Can other drugs interfere with the effects of the pill?"

Yes. Oral antibiotics, for example, can make the estrogen less effective.

THE MINI-PILL

The mini-pill (Nor-Q D) is a noncombination oral contraceptive that contains a synthetic progesterone and *no* estrogen. It acts by making the cervical mucus unpenetrable by sperm so the sperm can't connect with the egg. Although theoretically less effective than the standard combination pill, it is a reasonable choice for women over 40 who smoke or who can't take estrogen, especially since it can often stop hot flashes. The disadvantage is that about a third of women taking it have to endure a lot of spotting—breakthrough bleeding— which is annoying although nothing to worry about.

THE IUD: MAKING A COMEBACK

After virtually vanishing in the 1970s under a flurry of charges that it led to pelvic infections, sterility, and even death, the intrauterine device (IUD) has made a modest comeback and is now used by 5 percent of American women (compared to 15 to 25 percent of women in Europe). An IUD is a small plastic object that is inserted into the uterus in a ten-minute procedure performed under local anesthesia in the doctor's office and usually accompanied by a few days of antibiotics. If you are going to have any problems with it, they will probably occur in the first few days or weeks, when you may have some spotting and cramping. There is a small risk of infection for the first few months after insertion.

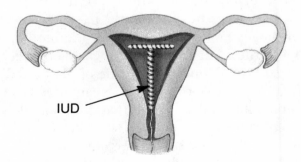

IUD

The IUD is a very effective contraceptive method that is often perfect for women who have only one partner and have finished having a family but do not want permanent sterilization. Many women choose it because they hesitate to take hormones but want a form of contraception that they don't have to think about every time they have intercourse. They want to put it in and forget about it.

Who Should *Not* Use the IUD

IUDs aren't for everyone, although they have been proven safe for hundreds of thousands of women world-wide. You should probably choose another form of contraception if you:

- Have a sexually transmitted infection
- Have had an ectopic pregnancy
- Are planning to have a child
- Are not in a mutually monogamous sexual relationship and plan to stay that way
- Have bleeding or coagulation disorders or anemia
- Are a diabetic

Currently available are two kinds of IUDs from which to choose. Progestasert, a flexible plastic T, slowly releases tiny amounts of progesterone that make the uterine lining unreceptive to a fertilized egg. It must be changed every year.

The Paragard, or Copper T, is made of plastic wrapped in copper wire. Changed once every six years, this IUD creates a mild noninfectious inflammation that does not allow an egg to become implanted.

You must check at least once a month to make sure the IUD is still in place by feeling for the string in your vagina and have it removed at menopause.

"Don't IUDs tend to become imbedded in the uterus and cause terrible problems?"

Rarely and then only when the IUD isn't changed on schedule. The Dalkan Shield—the one that cause the reputation of IUDs to nosedive—is no longer on the market.

"Why shouldn't you use an IUD if you and your partner are not mutually monogamous?"

Because it is possible that a sexually transmitted disease can infect your uterus and fallopian tubes more easily with an IUD in place. The more partners you have, the more you are exposed to multiple bacteria and viruses.

"Are IUDs advisable when you have fibroids?"

Not usually. Both fibroids and IUDs tend to increase menstrual bleeding. Besides, fibroids that impinge on the lining of the uterus could prevent the IUD from being positioned correctly.

NORPLANT: THE LATEST DEVELOPMENT

Norplant is the newest contraceptive option. It is probably the most effective reversible method of contraception available, so it can be a good choice for menstruating women in their forties or fifties who want birth control they don't have to think about every time they have intercourse but don't want to take the pill.

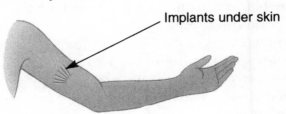
Implants under skin

Norplant works this way: Six little rods are implanted through a tiny incision just under the skin on the inside of the upper arm. The procedure, performed with local anesthesia, takes about ten minutes, requires no stitches, and is simply covered by a bandage for a day.

Once they are in place, you won't have to worry about getting pregnant for up to five years. The implants contain progestin (no estrogen) and release minute amounts of it slowly and steadily into the bloodstream, suppressing ovulation and blocking sperm by thickening the cervical mucus.

Advantages: Norplant is safe for smokers and its contraceptive effects are immediately reversible by removing it.

Disadvantages: It's expensive and harder to remove than to insert. In fact, there have been a number of complaints recently that removing it has caused pain, stress, and sometimes scarring. In most cases, however, the procedure is brief, simple, and painless. An added problem for some sensitive women are the typical side effects of progesterone such as weight gain, headaches, depression, and irregular menstrual bleeding.

DEPO-PROVERA

Although it's been used by millions of women around the world for more than twenty years, Depo-Provera was not approved for use in the United States until 1992. A long-acting synthetic progesterone taken by injection every three months, it acts by blocking ovulation and thickening the cervical mucus so sperm can't reach the egg.

Advantages: Because it doesn't contain estrogen, Depo-Provera is especially useful for women who can't take that hormone, but on the other hand, it doesn't give you estrogen's protective effects, either.

Disadvantages: Side effects are typical for progesterone:

weight gain, headaches, fatigue, irregular bleeding or spotting, irritability, depression. And because Depo-Provera is injected and lasts for three months, the side effects—if you have them—usually last for the same three months. Depo-Provera is not a good choice for women with a propensity for depression.

THE DIAPHRAGM

The diaphragm is tried-and-true and is 98 percent effective when correctly used. However, it has a fairly high failure rate of pregnancy prevention because using it correctly is sometimes easier said than done.

First, it must be inserted every time you have intercourse, requiring that you anticipate every sexual encounter or else interrupt the course of events. So very often the diaphragm is in the medicine cabinet when you need it most. Just this time, you persuade yourself, nothing will happen.

Second, to do its job it must fit properly or sperm can make their way around it. Besides, an ill-fitting diaphragm can be uncomfortable, even painful, and can cause urinary-tract infections. If you have gained or lost more than ten or fifteen pounds, or have had a baby, be sure to get the diaphragm refitted because your size may have changed. Diaphragms come in a variety of sizes, and yours must match that of your upper vagina or it doesn't do the job.

Third, the diaphragm must be inserted correctly if it is to block the sperm from reaching your cervix, uterus, and fallopian tubes. Get a lesson from your physician and then practice putting it in and taking it out. Get a second lesson, if necessary.

A diaphragm—a shallow rubber cup with flexible metal rims that fit snugly over the cervix—must *always* be used with spermicidal cream or jelly. The spermicide seals the edges (the fit is never 100 percent) and prevents sperm from circumventing the diaphragm.

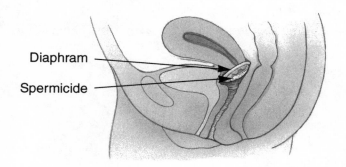

It's best to insert your diaphragm just before sexual activity. It is OK to put it in place in the morning if you are anticipating having sex at night, but you'll need to add spermicide just before intercourse or it will have lost some of its effectiveness. Afterwards, leave the diaphragm in place for at least six hours but no longer than twenty-four.

Advantages: The diaphragm doesn't interfere with your hormones or menstrual cycle and it causes no significant side effects. Used only when you need it, it is strictly temporary and can be a good choice if you have sex infrequently. Perhaps best of all, its use requires no cooperation from your partner.

Disadvantages: The failure rate for diaphragms is high when the diaphragm is not used correctly, however, or does not fit properly. It is considered messy and unaesthetic by some women, especially those who are squeamish about touching intimate parts of their own bodies. And it can cause vaginal irritation as well as bladder discomfort and infections, especially if it is too large or left in place for too long. Some women also have an allergic reaction to the rubber or the spermicide, causing irritation and recurrent urinary-tract infections.

"Why is a spermicide necessary and how should it be used?"

It seals the edges and kills the sperm on contact. Spread about a teaspoonful on the inside of the diaphragm, including the rim.

"Why isn't a lubricant good enough?"

Because it doesn't give you that extra margin of safety you need to keep enterprising sperm from making their way around it. *Never*, by the way, use petroleum jelly or any other oil-based lubricant with a diaphragm because it will eventually destroy the rubber.

"How often should a diaphragm be replaced?"

Take it with you to your annual gynecological checkup and let your doctor make that decision. It should last a couple of years if you take good care of it, which means washing it with mild soap and warm water after each use, drying it carefully, and dusting it with cornstarch (*not* talcum powder) before putting it back in its case. Check it for holes occasionally by filling it with water.

"Does a diaphragm protect you against infections or sexually transmitted diseases?"

Not at all. The *only* protection against infection and disease is a condom with spermicide. Besides, you may get more yeast and urinary-tract infections with a diaphragm because of local irritation.

SPERMICIDES

Contraceptive foams, creams, jellies, sponges, and suppositories are spermicides designed to be placed high in the vagina, where they kill sperm before they can enter the cervix. Best used in combination with condoms and diaphragms, alone they work about as well as the rhythm method, which shouldn't make you feel too secure.

The chemical nonoxynol 9, which is present in all spermicides, seems to offer a little protection against sexually transmitted diseases but don't count on it, especially when you use them alone without a condom. A recent study of women with many sex partners showed that use of a condom alone was more protective against infection than use of nonoxynol 9 alone. Always use the spermicide *and* a condom.

The contraceptive sponge is simply a synthetic sponge that has been impregnated with spermicide. Moistened with water, it is inserted in the back of the vagina. It has similar advantages and disadvantages as the diaphragm, although many women find it less messy and easier to insert and remove, and they like the fact that it is disposable. The major problem with the sponge is that it is less reliable than the diaphragm, especially for women who have had children.

Advantages: Spermicides are nonprescription, inexpensive, and easy to get.

Disadvantages: They have a higher failure rate, are messy, and must be reapplied before an additional act of intercourse. They must be applied no longer than a half hour before *each* act of intercourse, no matter how close together. Also they sometimes cause allergic reactions which can lead to vaginal irritation and urinary-tract infections.

CONDOMS

So many women are carrying male condoms around with them these days that "rubbers" could almost be considered a form of female contraception. The most frequently used barrier method in the United States today and the third most popular choice for married couples (after sterilization and the pill), condoms offer a low pregnancy rate when used by highly motivated couples who follow directions faithfully.

The condom is the *only* contraceptive choice when you have more than one sexual partner; when you are having sex with someone new; or when you are not absolutely certain (through testing) that your partner does not have AIDS, herpes, gonorrhea, chlamydia, HPV, or any other variety of sperm-transmitted disease that you don't want to get. Condoms, in fact, are the only contraceptive method that provides some protection against these diseases.

Condoms should be used with a spermicide *whether or not* you are already protected against pregnancy by oral contraceptives, an IUD, Norplant, or even sterilization. This maximizes the protection against sexually transmitted diseases. They must be put on *after* the penis is erect and *before* there is any contact between penis and vagina. Never use a condom twice; always use a new condom with *each* act of intercourse, vaginal, anal, or oral.

Use only latex (not natural-membrane or lambskin) condoms because they protect best against disease. Natural-membrane condoms have pores that are small enough to prevent passage of sperm but large enough to allow viruses to slip through.

Use only water-based lubricants or spermicides because other lubricants, such as petroleum jelly, vegetable shortening, body lotions, and oils, will destroy the latex.

The new female condom, marketed under the name Reality, is a lubricated polyurethane sheath with a polyurethane ring at each end. One ring is inserted into the vagina just past the pubic bone like a diaphragm, while the other remains outside the body surrounding the labia. One of its virtues is that it doesn't require the man's cooperation or permission and should offer similar advantages to the male condom. It is, however, more expensive, rather unaesthetic, and takes time to get used to.

Advantages: Condoms offer the best, although not perfect, protection against disease. They are cheap, available, and easy to use.

Disadvantages: They may destroy the spontaneity of sex because you must pause long enough to put them on an erect penis. Some men complain that they dampen sensation, but *you* are the one who is more likely to suffer the consequences of an STD or unintended pregnancy. Condoms deteriorate with time and heat, and have been known to break during ejaculation. Be careful not to tear them with your fingernails or teeth when opening the package.

STERILIZATION

Eleven million women have chosen permanent sterilization as their form of contraception; in fact, it is the most popular choice for married women over 40 in this country, where 700,000 tubal ligations and 500,000 vasectomies are performed each year. Reversal of sterilization is difficult and sometimes impossible, so consider this a very permanent procedure.

If you have decided you definitely do not want any—or any more—children, this may well be the way to go, as it is almost 100 percent effective. Besides, having your tubes tied greatly decreases your chances of ever developing ovarian cancer, according to recent research.

A tubal ligation, although not a major operation, is a surgical procedure. If not done during a cesarean delivery, it is usually performed in a laparoscopy when, through two small incisions, one in the belly button and the other at the pubic hairline, the fallopian tubes are severed, clamped, banded, or coagulated. This outpatient procedure takes about half an hour and is performed with local or light general anesthesia. You'll get back to normal activities within a week or so.

Advantages: Sterilization is permanent and extremely effective.

Disadvantages: It requires surgery and is not easily reversed. Sterilization sometimes causes shorter menstrual cycles and irregular bleeding, starting about two years after the operation. This is more common among women who have had irregular bleeding in the past and less common among those over 40. And if you have been sterilized, you are less likely to use condoms with new partners—a dangerous practice in today's social climate.

"Isn't it better for your husband to have a vasectomy?"

Vasectomies for a male partner are simpler, safer, and less expensive. Men are sometimes reluctant to consider vasectomy, however, because of recent reports of possible association with cancer and heart disease. There does not seem to be a connection between vasectomy and cardiovascular disease or testicular cancer. However, the waters are muddier when it comes to prostate cancer and some research has reported a weak epidemiological (but not causal) link between the two.

THE RHYTHM METHOD

Periodic sexual abstinence has been named the rhythm method, natural family planning, or Vatican roulette, depending on your point of view. The objective is to abstain from intercourse on the days that ovulation and fertilization are most likely to occur. Figuring out those days accurately is the big problem.

The calendar method takes the average length of your menstrual cycle and subtracts 14 to arrive at the approximate day of ovulation. Allowing for variations in the arrival of that day and for the length of time the sperm can survive in the cervical mucus results in blocking off seven days on either side of the predicted day.

To use the basal body temperature (BBT) method, you must take your temperature for three minutes before you get up every morning. Charting the temperatures will show that they usually rise a half-degree or more on the day after ovulation. Since the egg is not viable more than seventy-two hours after ovulation, the BBT method helps you detect the safe days after ovulation. But because it doesn't predict the safe days before ovulation, abstinence starts with the menstrual period.

The Billings' method requires that you become adept at detecting the presence of the slippery cervical mucus much like egg white that precedes ovulation and abstain from intercourse until that mucus disappears shortly after ovulation.

Advantages: No side effects and no risks.

Disadvantages: Because relatively long intervals of abstinence are required, pregnancy rates are usually rather high. If you are highly motivated, the extra effort and uncertainty are reasonable tradeoffs.

Chapter 10

HAVING A BABY: ORCHESTRATING A LATE PREGNANCY

IF YOU ARE AMONG the one in every five women in the United States who has her first child after age 35, you are part of a rapidly growing group. Late pregnancies have increased 50 percent in just the last ten years. In fact, 35 isn't considered late anymore, as it becomes more and more common for women to wait until they're 40 or so to decide they want to have a first child or to complete a family.

The reasons may be financial, educational, professional, or simply personal. Sociologists point to the availability of effective birth control and safe and legal abortion, combined with the cultural influences of the sexual revolution, the growing numbers of working women, feminism, and increased independence for women. But whatever the reasons, this is a generation that has consciously postponed having children. Three times as many women are having their first baby after age 35 as twenty years ago.

Getting pregnant the old-fashioned way, however, may not always be easy. That's because now you are at the eleventh hour of your reproductive life. Your lifetime supply of egg follicles is running out, and your production of estrogen is diminishing.

The limited supply of eggs is believed to be the chief reason that fertility decreases with age. In addition, the remaining eggs get older and less fertile with each passing year while, at the same time, the uterus may become less receptive to a pregnancy. The truth is that the older you are, the slimmer your chances of conceiving and maintaining a pregnancy. Starting at around age 37, fertility definitely declines with age and, statistically, drops precipitously after the age of 41.

The chances of miscarriage and birth defects also increase as you grow older because the uterus gradually becomes less able to support an embryo, while the percentage of chromosomally abnormal or damaged embryos rises from an incidence of about two in ten at age 40 to four or five in ten at 45.

But all of these disheartening statistics don't mean *you* cannot become pregnant and have a healthy baby if you are over 40. Statistics are interesting, but they are generalities about whole populations and don't necessarily apply to you. Women today are having babies long after their prime childbearing years and, with the help of amazing new techniques, even long after menopause.

If you want to have a baby now, don't be overly discouraged by the numbers. Obviously, some women are biologically younger than others at the same chronological age and have ovaries that function well for a longer time than average. Besides, if you do get pregnant, no matter how hard it is for other women to achieve their goal, *you* are 100 percent pregnant.

Pregnancies in women over 40 account for 1 percent of all pregnancies in the United States today. Ironically, 80 percent of them are unplanned.

"Why is it harder for me to get pregnant now?"

Mainly because, by the time you have reached your late thirties or early forties, you are running out of viable eggs. Eggs are not replenished like skin, muscle, or bone. A woman is born with all the eggs she will ever have and enters puberty with about 200,000 microscopic oocytes per ovary. During each menstrual cycle, the pituitary gland releases enough FSH (follicle-stimulating hormone) to stimulate the development of about 1,000 eggs. After two weeks of growth, the largest egg is released or ovulated, while the rest are reabsorbed into the connective tissue of the ovary never to develop again.

After you have gone through thirty years or so of monthly ovulations, the vast majority of your eggs have been released or reabsorbed. At the same time, those that remain gradually lose their ability to be fertilized, to implant in the uterus, and to develop into normal fetuses.

"I have been controlling my fertility for more than fifteen years with oral contraceptives, but now I'd like to have a child. Will using the pill for so long spoil my chances?"

Most likely you will start ovulating again in three to six months after you quit the pill if you have no other problems and haven't reached menopause, so your chances will be as good as ever at your age. In rare cases, however, the pituitary gland continues to be suppressed after the pills are discontinued and may need stimulation by fertility drugs.

HOW LATE CAN I WAIT?

Studies have shown that only about half of all women have the natural biological ability to conceive at 41 and only one in ten can manage to become pregnant at age 45. Therefore, it obviously makes sense to start as early as possible and not to wait too long before seeking expert help. Although infertility is broadly defined as the failure to conceive after twelve months, six fruitless months are probably long enough for women in this age group to wait before looking for other answers.

If you want to have a baby and it doesn't seem to be happening in the usual way, what can you do about it? You can be treated by a specialist in infertility who will use one or more of many sophisticated techniques to help you conceive and then hold on to the fetus. Doctors today can manipulate virtually every aspect of the reproductive cycle, enhancing your own reproductive capabilities and/or bypassing your particular barriers to fertility.

We recommend that you research infertility treatment thoroughly before deciding whether to go ahead with it. It is time-consuming, often discouraging or even heartbreaking, and it can be very costly. Your doctor will certainly give you his or her best medical opinion about your chances of success, but in the end it is you who must decide whether the odds are too small or the expenses too great.

Be a careful consumer. Check out the qualifications, experience, success rates, and personalities of the physicians, medical groups, or clinics you are considering, perhaps seeking guidance from the American Fertility Society or Resolve, the national consumer infertility organization.

And then, once into infertility treatment, you must decide when it makes sense to stop if it isn't working. Sometimes that's the most difficult decision of all.

For information and referrals:

American Fertility Society
1209 Montgomery Highway
Birmingham, Alabama 35216

or

Resolve
1310 Broadway
Somerville, Massachusetts
02144-1731
617-623-0744

"Are there tests to determine whether there is any real possibility of getting pregnant naturally or with outside help?"

At this moment, the best way to know whether you have enough eggs and estrogen to make conception possible is to measure your FSH level for clues about your "ovarian age." The level of FSH (follicle-stimulating hormone) circulating in the bloodstream gradually rises as your estrogen level declines, so it provides a logical way to predict the possibility of pregnancy.

In general, if your FSH measures less than 10 mIU/ml, you can get pregnant almost as easily as a younger woman. Your chances decrease as the FSH level goes up and by the time it reaches 25 mIU/ml, pregnancy is pretty much out of the question (unless you receive a donated egg) because you are on the brink of menopause.

"How is FSH measured?"

A blood sample is taken on one of the first three days of the menstrual cycle when every woman's FSH level is at its very lowest point. If at this lowest point the FSH level is over 25 mIU/ml—or anywhere near it—then you know your ovaries probably cannot be stimulated to produce healthy eggs.

"If I am having perfectly normal periods at age 47, doesn't that mean I could get pregnant?"

Certainly, although it's not very likely. With normal periods, it is always possible to get pregnant; that's why doctors always recommend using birth control until you are certifiably menopausal if you don't want to have a baby. However, at 47, a successful pregnancy is rare and the risk of miscarriage very high.

"What are the infertility treatments for older women today?"

A combination of fertility drugs with intrauterine insemination, IVF, GIFT, or ZIFT (which are explained below). But once you have reached about 43, these techniques are usually unsuccessful because of the age-related biological changes in your remaining eggs (known in the trade as "the decline in oocyte quality").

On the other hand, if the age of your eggs is the major factor that causes infertility as you grow older, the obvious answer is to use a younger egg—in other words, egg donation, the very newest option. Women older than 40 are just as successful at having babies with donated eggs as younger women and, in fact, egg donation has become the most successful of all infertility treatments for women of any age. Indeed, the older woman who receives a donated egg that is then fertilized and placed in the uterus achieves a "per cycle pregnancy rate" that rivals that of the highest natural fertility at any age.

Even women past menopause can now have babies with the help of this new technique. In a recent study of fourteen postmenopausal women ages 50 to 59 who tried this procedure, eight became pregnant. The oldest was 55.

INFERTILITY TREATMENTS

The treatment of infertility has made enormous progress in the last few years because of a series of remarkable advances in assisted reproductive technology, or ART. This technology combines the use of fertility drugs—hormonal therapy—with artificial insemination using any of a group of techniques: intrauterine insemination (IUI), in vitro fertilization (IVF), gamete intrafallopian transfer (GIFT), zygote intrafallopian transfer (ZIFT), or oocyte (egg) donation.

FERTILITY DRUGS

Fertility drugs, forms of hormone therapy, are designed to trick the ovaries into producing eggs, sometimes many eggs in a single cycle, by stimulating your own hormones to do their assigned jobs more efficiently or by replacing them entirely with "outside" hormones.

Clomiphene, marketed under the brand names Clomid and Serophene and used for the treatment of fertility problems for more than twenty-five years, is an agent that increases your own hormone production. Taken by tablet, clomiphene works by making the pituitary gland produce large quantities of FSH. The FSH in turn stimulates ovulation—in fact, sometimes accomplishing its purpose so well that it results in the release of two or more eggs, giving a woman on clomiphene a 10 percent chance of carrying twins.

Side Effects: Temporary and harmless, clomiphene's side effects can be bothersome or even unnerving if you don't know what to expect. They include the following:

1. Hot flashes, just like those you may get at menopause, because of an increased FSH level.

2. Mild disturbances in vision, noticeable mainly in the dark, that make colors seem to smear or trail behind objects when you move your head.

3. Mood swings, ranging from irritability to heightened emotional responses, lack of concentration, and "spaciness." In fact, you may feel like you are suffering from a bad case of PMS.

4. Ovarian pain or sensitivity around the time of ovulation, probably because the ovary is stretched when multiple eggs are stimulated to grow all at once.

5. Ovarian cysts—not the same as the ovarian cysts that require surgery, but merely the small fluid-filled follicles that do not burst open, releasing an egg at the time of ovulation and then continue to grow. Almost always symptomless, they usually vanish after the next menstrual period and rarely require treatment.

Pergonal and *Metrodin* are powdered forms of the human pituitary hormone FSH (follicle-stimulating hormone). They are mixed with sterile water and taken by daily intramuscular injections. Unlike clomiphene, these drugs bypass the pituitary gland and stimulate the ovary directly. And they usually prompt the release of many eggs at a time, increasing the odds of conception. Another advantage over naturally occuring hormones is that they allow precise control of the timing of ovulation, making possible such advanced procedures as IUI, IVF, or GIFT.

A cycle stimulated by Pergonal or Metrodin must be carefully and regularly monitored to make sure the ovaries are stimulated neither too little nor too much. Visualization by transvaginal ultrasound allows the number of eggs to be counted and their maturity estimated, while blood tests for estrogen level indicate the degree of ovarian stimulation and the readiness of the eggs for release.

When the eggs are mature, an intramuscular injection of human chorionic gonadotrophin (hCG), a hormone normally produced in huge quantities in early pregnancy, triggers ovulation within about thirty-six hours. The thirty-six-hour interval gives time for planning intercourse, insemination, or retrieval of eggs for IVF or GIFT. This hormone is also sometimes used with clomiphene to time intercourse or artificial insemination.

Because of the large number of eggs usually produced when Pergonal or Metrodin is used, a woman who becomes pregnant with its help has a 20 percent chance of carrying twins, a 5 percent chance of triplets, and a 1 percent chance of quadruplets. But the risks of losing the pregnancy or having very premature babies increase when there are more than three embryos, so pregnancy reduction—the removal of the extra embryos—is the usual recommendation.

Side Effects: Pergonal or Metrodin treatment often results in mild abdominal bloating and water retention in the week after ovulation. These symptoms are both transient and benign. If the ovaries are overstimulated, however, you may have nausea, abdominal distention, rapid weight gain, and swollen ovaries, a situation that requires prompt medical treatment or maybe even hospitalization for careful monitoring of your salt and fluid balance. This occurs less than 1 percent of the time.

INTRAUTERINE INSEMINATION (IUI)

In this procedure, a small amount of concentrated sperm, first "washed" to remove most of the seminal plasma that surrounds it, is placed in the uterus through a thin plastic catheter that is passed through the vagina and cervix. Usually painless, the IUI procedure takes only a few minutes to accomplish.

IUI is almost always used in combination with a fertility drug—clomiphene or Pergonal—to stimulate ovulation followed by an hCG injection to trigger the release of an egg. The timing of the IUI is determined with the help of vaginal ultrasound, previous cycle lengths, BBT temperature graphs, or urinary LH correlation kits. In a natural menstrual cycle, when the egg is mature, it uses estrogen to trigger the release of luteinizing hormone (LH) from the pituitary gland. The LH can be detected with a home kit twenty-four to forty-eight hours before ovulation. If IUI is successful in producing a pregnancy, it usually happens within the first six menstrual cycles.

IN VITRO FERTILIZATION (IVF)

In vitro fertilization is designed to make it easier for the egg and the sperm to meet successfully by taking essential reproductive events out of the body and performing them in vitro. *In vitro* means "in glass," as in a test tube (hence the term "test tube baby"). Mature eggs are removed from the ovaries, fertilized with sperm in a laboratory dish, and then the resulting embryo is implanted into the uterus.

IVF, first used to treat women with absent or damaged fallopian tubes, is used today for any kind of infertility, from "unexplained" infertility to male infertility, low sperm count, cervical problems, and endometriosis. It has supplanted most other treatments to become the ultimate option—except for egg donation—because it allows the specialist to bypass most of the important barriers to a pregnancy.

Although there are many IVF programs throughout the country today, each differing in minor ways, all use the following four steps:

1. *Ovarian stimulation.* One of the earliest breakthroughs in IVF technique was the realization that the quickest way to increase the chances of pregnancy was to increase the number of eggs to be fertilized and returned to the body. Many ways of achieving "superovulation" are practiced, but most IVF centers in the United States use either Pergonal or Metrodin or a combination of both.

The development of the follicles is closely followed by observing their growth with transvaginal ultrasound and measuring their ability to produce estrogen. When the eggs are big enough, they are ready for egg retrieval.

2. *Egg retrieval.* In the natural menstrual cycle, mature follicles rupture (that's ovulation) and the eggs are expelled from the surface of the ovary into the fallopian tube. During IVF, the eggs are removed just before ovulation. Here's how it is done: After you are sedated, a speculum is used to expand the vagina, and a thin needle is passed through the back wall of the vagina up to the ovaries, all accomplished with the guidance of transvaginal ultrasound. As the doctor watches the procedure on the screen of the ultrasound machine, the needle punctures the follicle and, with gentle suction, carefully removes the egg along with the follicular fluid.

One by one, the eggs are placed in a sterile container and examined under the microscope by a cell biologist or embryologist. If they are judged normal in shape and development, they are ready for fertilization.

3. *Fertilization.* Now the eggs and fresh "washed" sperm are mixed together for fertilization. When fertilization has indeed taken place and the eggs, now called embryos, are beginning to undergo cell division, they are graded and prepared for transfer to the uterus.

4. *Embryo transfer.* One to three days after the eggs are retrieved, up to four healthy embryos are inserted into the uterus with a thin plastic tube that is passed through the cervix. To be sure there is enough progesterone to develop the uterine lining for implantation of at least one of the embryos, injections of progesterone or hCG are given for the next two weeks.

Serum hCG (pregnancy hormone) levels are measured ten to fourteen days after the transfer for the first indications of whether any of the embryos have implanted. If they have been successful, repeated measurements of hCG will show if the pregnancy is proceeding normally until the number of developing embryos can be counted via transvaginal ultrasound two weeks later.

GAMETE INTRAFALLOPIAN TRANSFER (GIFT)

GIFT is a more sophisticated variation of the basic IVF procedure and usually produces a slightly higher pregnancy rate. Everything is the same until the eggs, or "gametes," are to be retrieved. Then, instead of being withdrawn from the ovaries with a needle through the vagina, they are removed through the abdominal wall via laparoscopy. The eggs combined with the prepared sperm are immediately placed inside a catheter, then transferred to a fallopian tube, where fertilization occurs naturally. Of course, this method is possible only when the fallopian tubes are not blocked or damaged.

ZYGOTE INTRAFALLOPIAN TRANSFER (ZIFT)

This is the latest variation on the IVF-GIFT technique. With this even more sophisticated method, the follicles are stimulated and the eggs extracted from the ovaries transvaginally, as with IVF, but now the freshly fertilized eggs—zygotes—are placed into the fallopian tubes during a laparoscopy after they have reached the embryo stage. ZIFT thus combines the advantage of knowing that fertilization has truly taken place with GIFT's more natural placement directly into the fallopian tubes.

EGG DONATION

Is egg donation appropriate for you? It may well be your answer if your ovaries have been damaged or removed because of endometriosis, infection, or tumors; if they have stopped functioning properly; if your eggs did not manage to be fertilized with IVF; or if, because of age-related changes, other treatment simply hasn't worked.

Here's how it's done. After the egg donor has been screened and selected, the menstrual cycles of the donor and recipient are synchronized with the use of Synarel (a nasal spray) or Lupron (an injection) so that the recipient's uterine receptivity is maximized at the same time as the donor's eggs become mature. The donor receives injections of FSH (Pergonal or Metrodin) to stimulate the release of many eggs at once, while the recipient gets twice-a-week injections of estrogen to prepare the lining of her uterus.

Several mature eggs are retrieved, fertilized in the laboratory, and transferred into the recipient's uterus by a small plastic tube passed through the vagina and cervix. The hormonal needs of an early pregnancy are met by daily administration of progesterone and continuation of the twice-a-week estrogen injections. A pregnancy test two weeks later lets you know whether you have achieved your goal.

"How is the donor chosen?"

The major qualifications for the egg donor are that she is young, preferably under the age of 30, and healthy. If she has been pregnant before, that is reassuring but not an absolute prerequisite. She may be a family member, a friend, or someone provided by an independent recruitment service that finds and screens suitable candidates. The customary screening fee to the agency is about $2,500 while the fee to the donor is usually about the same.

All egg donors, family or otherwise, are screened and counseled concerning the medical, legal, and psychological issues. The donor's medical history is closely investigated and blood tests are performed for hepatitis, syphilis, HIV, and cytomegalovirus. And before going ahead she signs a legal contract, agreeing to give up all rights to any offspring resulting from the procedure.

You, as the recipient, must assume all legal responsibilities for the outcome of the donation, including medical complications of the pregnancy or the child. And you too are psychologically screened and counseled.

"What are the chances of success?"

Excellent, about 50 percent per cycle. That's higher than IVF or GIFT pregnancy rates *and* higher than the maximum "natural" fertility rate of about 33 percent per cycle.

"How much does it cost?"

Altogether, including the donor's fee and the costs of the screening and the procedure itself, anywhere from $7,500 to $15,000.

"As a woman of 42, what are my chances of getting pregnant with IVF?"

Under the most favorable circumstances, IVF pregnancy rates rival those of normal fertility. Unfortunately, being over 40 means the circumstances are not the most favorable since success rates decrease significantly with every passing year. For one thing, you are now less likely to respond to the stimulation of fertility drugs with large numbers of eggs and may develop only one or two. In addition, miscarriage rates in IVF pregnancies for older women can be brutally high.

You have, therefore, a tough decision to make, especially since IVF is expensive, time-consuming, and stressful. The bottom line is that, with IVF, the pregnancy rate is 10 to 15 percent per cycle for women at 40. But then the rate falls off so rapidly that very few women over the age of 42 can realistically expect to achieve pregnancy and would be well advised to turn to egg donation or adoption instead.

On the other hand, IVF also maximizes your odds over the shortest length of time. So it is a close call that depends on whether you have the money and the emotional and physical stamina it may require.

"I had menopause two years ago at age 41. Is there any possibility that the fertility drugs could allow me to conceive?"

No. When your FSH level is way up and you are definitely menopausal, you no longer produce much estrogen and whatever leftover egg follicles remain have become resistant to the stimulation of the drugs. The purpose of fertility drugs is to add to or stimulate the production of FSH, and you are already making plenty.

On the other hand, if your FSH level has not risen to menopausal heights and you were not ovulating for some other reason, then the drugs are definitely worth a try.

"One thing that bothers me about taking fertility drugs is the idea of having to abort some of the embryos if too many eggs are implanted. I don't think I could deal with that. Are there any alternatives?"

No, except to take your chances. But remember that for older women the possibility of conceiving triplets or even more babies as the result of using fertility drugs is much lower than it is for younger women. "Pregnancy reduction," which looks and feels like an amniocentesis, certainly has its moral and emotional complications and it is a decision that few women approach without doubt and trepidation. But keep in mind that its purpose is to enhance your safety and to increase the chances that the remaining embryos will survive.

Today triplets usually do quite well, matching twins in survival and outcome, although they will definitely be born prematurely and small. The pregnancy is usually complicated by lots of bed rest, monitoring for premature labor, hospitalization in the third trimester, and a cesarean delivery.

Pregnancy with more than triplets, however, is fraught with difficulty and should be undertaken only under the care of the most sophisticated and experienced obstetrical and pediatric team possible.

"Can fertility drugs cause cancer?"

A recent study proposes that fertility drugs could raise the risk of ovarian cancer, but the small number of cancers among the 12 million women who have taken these drugs and the stable rate of ovarian cancer despite such increasing use of these drugs suggest that this is probably not true. It's long been known that any woman who has never been pregnant has an increased risk of developing ovarian cancer. And it is "biologically plausible" that the additional ovulations induced by fertility drugs can make the ovaries more susceptible to cancer or that the higher levels of FSH encouraged by the drugs can overstimulate the ovaries, thereby leading to cancer.

However, women who have taken fertility drugs and then became pregnant have not shown a higher risk of ovarian cancer. So what may be true is that women who have never conceived despite the assistance of fertility drugs may have some intrinsic abnormality that prevents pregnancy *and* puts them at higher risk for cancer. See Chapter 14 for more about ovarian cancer.

"I am 41 and have been trying to have a baby for over two years. I have a couple of very large fibroids and I am wondering if they may be the cause of my difficulty."

Fibroids are rarely a cause of infertility unless they are extremely large—they are more likely to cause a miscarriage.

STAYING PREGNANT

Getting pregnant is half the battle. The other half is *staying* pregnant for nine months or close to it and giving birth to a healthy baby. Fortunately, this is a job that is only a little more complicated for older women. The major problem occurs during the very early days or weeks of the pregnancy, when chances of miscarriage are the highest for all women but especially for those in their forties.

Surprisingly, very little is known about miscarriages and even less about how to prevent them. We do know that they occur in at least 15 percent of women whose pregnancies have been confirmed. We don't know, however, how many fertilized eggs never implant, or implant so fleetingly that they don't even delay the following menstrual period, but it is probable that this undetected loss occurs in half of all fertilizations.

Most of the time, an early miscarriage means that the pregnancy would not have produced a healthy baby because a high percentage of eggs, perhaps even one in three, is not perfectly normal. That's little comfort, of course, if you are the one to whom it happens, but whatever your age, chromosomal defects are almost always a matter of chance and so may never happen again.

WHY MISCARRIAGES?

Most miscarriages result from chromosomally abnormal embryos and tend to occur with increasing frequency with age. At puberty, a young girl has approximately 400,000 egg follicles divided between her two ovaries, but by the age of 40, she has only 5,000 to 10,000 left, making the chances of ovulating an abnormal egg more and more likely. Genetic defects occur in only about 15 percent of pregnancies before 35, but rise to approximately 25 percent by age 40 and as high as 50 percent by age 45.

In 99 out of 100 cases, however, abnormal embryos fail to implant or are expelled, usually within only a few weeks of conception. That leaves only about 1 in 100 pregnancies with abnormal chromosomes surviving into the second trimester, when the defect can be detected by amniocentesis or chorionic villus sampling (CVS).

For referrals and information on
genetic counseling, contact your local
March of Dimes chapter or:
March of Dimes
Birth Defects Foundation
1275 Mamaroneck Avenue
White Plains, New York 10605

THE NEED FOR PRENATAL TESTING

As you get older, your chances of having a child with a chromosomal problem such as Down's syndrome increase significantly. That's why prenatal tests are always recommended if you are over 35 and strongly suggested if you are over 40, to allay your fears if all is well or to give you the option of ending the pregnancy and trying again if it isn't. The risk of having a child with a chromosomal abnormality increases from about half of 1 percent at 35 to 1.5 percent at 40, to 5 percent at age 45.

Amniocentesis The best-known test for abnormal fetal cells, this is usually performed between the fifteenth and eighteenth weeks of a pregnancy. The fourteenth week is considered the earliest it may be done safely. Using ultrasound, the physician views the fetus on a TV monitor as it floats inside a sac filled with amniotic fluid within the uterus. Then, after injecting a local anesthetic and while carefully watching the position of the fetus, the doctor inserts a long needle through the abdominal and uterine walls into the amniotic sac and withdraws a small amount of fluid. This fluid contains fetal cells whose chromosomes can be carefully examined and counted under a microscope.

The advantage of amniocentesis is that it is slightly safer than CVS (see below), with a lower chance of inadvertently precipitating a miscarriage. It also allows for the measurement of fetal proteins and hormones to help detect the presence of spinal bifida or other nervous system abnormalities. The risk of fetal injury is practically zero. The results are available within about three weeks.

Chorionic Villus Sampling (CVS)   This test may be performed as early as the ninth week of pregnancy. Again, ultrasound provides a clear view of the fetus. Then a speculum is placed in the vagina just as it is for a routine pelvic examination and a thin hollow tube is carefully passed through the cervix and into the uterus, where it extracts a few of the placenta's hairlike projections, called chorionic villi, which contain the same genetic material as the fetus. The sample is then analyzed, with results in only a week or so.

Which way to go? Amniocentesis is slightly safer for a normal pregnancy because it precipitates fewer miscarriages (its risk is .5 percent vs. 1 to 2 percent for CVS), while CVS gives earlier and quicker results and so it is slightly safer and less emotionally traumatic for the mother if she decides to terminate an abnormal pregnancy.

"Why does it take so interminably long to get the results of an amniocentesis? And why are CVS results quicker?"

With amniocentesis, the cells found in the amniotic fluid must first be cultured and grown in the laboratory. That takes time. With CVS, you have a sample of tissue that may be microscopically examined immediately.

OTHER CAUSES OF MISCARRIAGE

Although abnormalities of the embryo are the usual reason for losing a pregnancy early on, there is constant debate among medical experts about the possible effects of other factors.

- *Hormonal imbalance.* Low progesterone production resulting in an underdeveloped uterine lining is thought to be a possible reason for miscarriage. Called *luteal phase defect*, this is a problem that becomes more common with age. It has been found that when the progesterone level in the blood is below 15 mIU/ml, the pregnancy is usually lost. Treatment commonly includes raising the progesterone level with fertility drugs or progesterone suppositories.
- *Uterine or cervical problems.* If you have had repeated miscarriages, especially later in your pregnancies, the problem may be found in an incompetent cervix (a cervix that is unable to stay closed and "hold" the pregnancy), a uterus that is partly divided by a wall or *septum*, or a uterus whose space has been usurped by a very large fibroid. Possible solutions include surgical closure of the cervix or removal of the septum or the fibroids.
- *Infections.* Although their role in precipitating miscarriage is still unclear, it is considered possible for an acute infectious illness to cause the loss of a pregnancy. Such infections include salmonella, measles, rubella, chicken pox, herpes, syphilis, toxoplasmosis, and cytomegalovirus. Whether the presence of any other benign microorganism called a *mycoplasma* (urea plasma) causes miscarriage is still open to debate.
- *Immune system problems.* The newest—and least understood—ideas about miscarriage are related to a malfunctioning of the immune system, when antibodies are formed to fight against the body's own tissues. Blood tests can reveal the presence of two auto-antibodies, either

of which are thought to cause miscarriage. The first is *anticardiolipin antibody*, which can cause an acceleration in blood clotting near the implantation site of the embryo. The second is *lupus anticoagulant*, which raises the risk of an abnormality in blood clotting, interfering with implantation as well as the development of the placenta. The usual treatment for these problems is a small daily dose of aspirin, sometimes combined with a low dose of heparin, to combat the tendency of the blood to clot too readily.

• *Environmental causes.* We are subjected to multiple health hazards from a contaminated environment, ranging from air pollution and toxic wastes to hormone-treated meat and pesticide-adulterated produce to more than 77,000 different chemicals commonly used by industry. Although evidence points to higher rates of miscarriage as a result of exposure to these substances, little has yet been scientifically proven. Nevertheless, it is certainly wise to do your best when you are pregnant to avoid as many of them as possible, including alcohol, all unnecessary drugs (prescription or otherwise), nicotine, paints, and solvents. Other practical suggestions are to wear a protective apron if you must have dental X-rays and use a low-emission computer monitor. Stay out of hot tubs and saunas because excessive heat has been linked to fetal damage.

"Is it hazardous to my own health to have a baby at 43?"

A healthy woman, even having her first baby, is in no more danger than anyone else simply because she is over 40, except for a slightly higher than normal risk of developing a transient form of diabetes (gestational diabetes) or heightened blood pressure and toxemia during the pregnancy. And, of course, by the time any of us reaches the age of 40 or 45, we may have acquired medical problems that could be complicated by a pregnancy.

"Are there any special risks of a late pregnancy for the baby other than Down's syndrome?"

No, except for a slightly higher chance of delivering an under-weight baby. So if the results of an amniocentesis or CVS are good, you face no greater risk of bearing a child with a birth defect than a younger woman.

"Are older mothers more likely to have cesarean sections?"

Yes, there's a two- to threefold increased risk of a cesarean. But this is related to your age only because both you and your physician are especially eager to have a successful outcome and therefore have a lower threshold for deciding on a surgical delivery. If there is a marginal risk of some sort—perhaps a breech baby or the possibility of a moderate amount of disproportion between mother and baby—most doctors would perform a cesarean in order to avoid taking even a very small chance that something might go wrong. Their decision is usually based on the fact that you do not have many years of childbearing capacity ahead of you.

Chapter 11

YOUR VAGINA: VAGINITIS AND OTHER CONCERNS

VAGINITIS IS A CATCHALL TERM for several different types of inflammations, irritations, and common infections that are almost every woman's lot, especially as the vagina starts to show its age. With the passage of time two things happen. First, with the decrease in estrogen production the lining of your vagina becomes dryer and thinner, making it more easily inflamed and irritated and, as a result, more vulnerable to infection.

Second, the pH of the vagina, normally acidic during your younger years, becomes much more alkaline as your estrogen level declines. A less acidic vagina is more hospitable to harmful organisms and, at the same time, less inviting to the normal friendly flora whose job it is to defend you against them.

If you add sexual activity, which exposes you to vaginal trauma as well as to outside bacteria, you have a perfect setup for vaginitis.

Vaginal burning, itching, discharge, irritation, and inflammation are all symptoms of vaginitis, which comes in four basic varieties, each quite different and with its own specific treatment.

WHAT YOU CAN DO *NOW*

Seriously consider hormone replacement therapy if you have had menopause and suffer from never-ending infections and irritations. It is your only hope for restoring the tissues to a state that's not so attractive to bacteria and other malevolent organisms. Vaginal estrogen cream may be all that's required.

Also, never ignore infections because they usually get worse and more tenacious without treatment. If you treat them right away as soon as the symptoms appear, you will have a better chance of clearing them up fast. Chronic cases can be very stubborn. Also you must identify your ailment promptly because it is entirely possible, given our current sexual climate, that you could have contracted something more serious than vaginitis (see Chapter 8). Make sure your doctor makes the appropriate tests to determine which infection you have before prescribing treatment.

Then:

- Ask if your sexual partner should be medicated too, since many infections are passed back and forth and so never are eradicated for good.
- Use a lubricant during sexual intercourse to reduce the friction and help the tissues to stretch.
- Choose your bed partners carefully. Insist on a condom with a man you don't know well or totally trust. Never take chances on the ailments described in Chapter 8.
- Never use tampons for a discharge or a light flow. Use them only on days of heavy flow and then change them frequently.
- If you have recurrent vaginitis, don't use tampons at all until you've been symptom-free for at least three months.
- Avoid douches (except for a vinegar or boric acid douche), feminine hygiene sprays, deodorant tampons, bath gels, bubble baths, and perfumed soap, all of which can be irritating and drying.

- Keep yourself scrupulously clean, using only mild nonperfumed soap and water.
- Stay out of whirlpools and hot tubs, even your own, if you have a tendency to get vaginitis.
- Step up your consumption of vitamin C, which seems to help some women fight vaginal inflammation.

ATROPHIC VAGINITIS

When your vagina lining, suffering from an estrogen deficiency, has lost its thick protective layer of cornified cells, much of its former ability to lubricate itself, and its "rugal folds" which allow it to expand and contract during sex, it becomes thin, dry, irritable, tight, and nonelastic—in other words, it is now atrophic. That makes it subject to a chronic inflammation so common it has a name: atrophic vaginitis. This is a condition, not an infection, but it sets the vagina up for injury, trauma, bleeding, and pain, especially after intercourse, and makes it less able to fight off many nasty infectious organisms.

WHAT YOU CAN DO ABOUT ATROPHIC VAGINITIS

The ideal remedy for atrophic vaginitis is hormone replacement therapy—it's the only way to restore these fragile tissues to their formerly functional state. The estrogen may be taken by pill or patch, in which case it also provides protection for your bones and your heart. And/or it may be applied locally in the form of estrogen cream. Whatever route, it will rejuvenate your vagina in a hurry. For details, see Chapter 3.

If you can't or don't wish to take estrogen, try using a vaginal nonhormone moisturizer that hydrates the cells of vaginal lining and allows them to build up a continually moist protective layer. It also lowers the pH of the vagina, making it less inviting to unfriendly bacteria. Again, the details can be found in Chapters 3 and 6.

YEAST INFECTIONS

Yeast infections (a.k.a. monilia, candida albicans, or candidiasis) are the most common form of vaginal infection, afflicting half of all women at some time in their lives. Yeast is a fungus that is a perfectly normal inhabitant of the vagina as well as other parts of the body and, in fact, the environment. In small numbers it causes no problems. But when the organism is encouraged by circumstances to run rampant and proliferate in your reproductive tract, it can make your life miserable.

If you have a yeast infection, you'll know it because of intense itching and burning around the entrance to the vagina and very often a thick white discharge that may look like cottage cheese.

Nobody knows why some women are especially susceptible to an overgrowth of yeast, but we do know the circumstances that increase your chances of getting it. One of the major instigators is the use of broad-spectrum antibiotics (tetracycline is one of the chief offenders, even if you use it only on your skin; so is ampicillin), which destroy the lactobacillus—the friendly bacteria that normally protect the vagina from just such invasions.

Another is a lot of sugary foods in your diet. Yeast apparently likes high blood sugar, the reason why diabetics are especially prone to this problem. Other triggers include steroid treatment, the use of oral contraceptives, and pregnancy, which causes an inviting buildup of starch in the vaginal cells. Because yeast is happiest in dark, moist, heated environments, these infections are most common in summer.

One of the best things that's ever come along for women

is the development of medications for yeast that may now be purchased over the counter, without a prescription. Many women have three or four yeast infections a year, and it's a burden to continually run to their doctors for prescriptions.

Be sure, of course, that your diagnosis is correct before you use them. If you are not certain that yeast is what's ailing you or if the symptoms aren't clearcut, go to your doctor for an evaluation. It is quite possible that you have something else that is much more serious and damaging—not something you want to leave untreated.

WHAT YOU CAN DO ABOUT YEAST INFECTIONS

- *See your gynecologist.* Although after a while you will readily recognize a yeast infection's symptoms, if you have never had one before or you are at all uncertain, go to your doctor. An accurate diagnosis is important. What works for one vaginal infection doesn't work for another. The doctor should look at a smear of your vaginal secretions under a microscope, where the fungus may be seen in great numbers, or make a culture of it for evaluation by a microbiology laboratory. If you have a yeast infection, the doctor will then recommend a nonprescription drug (see below) or prescribe an antifungal cream or suppository.

  Go to your doctor, too, if you get many yeast infections a year. Although these fungal infections usually respond very quickly to treatment, some women get them again and again and may need longer-term treatment, such as a systemic antifungal medication.
- *Use an over-the-counter antifungal medication.* These include Monistat, Gyne-Lotrimin, Femstat, Vagistat, and Mycelex-G. Most are to be applied for seven days, although some double-strength preparations call for only three days of treatment and one offers relief in a single dose. Most women find they need at least seven days of medication to

get rid of a yeast infection and some require an additional seven-day course of treatment to ban the bug. If you have followed the directions faithfully and the medication doesn't seem to be doing the job in the allotted time, go to your doctor for a culture.

• *Use an antifungal medication prophylactically.* In other words, use it to *prevent* infection when you take antibiotics. Start using the medication the day you begin taking the antibiotics and continue until the antibiotic treatment is completed.

• *Eat yogurt.* This inexpensive folk remedy may be as effective as its long-time proponents have always claimed, according to a recent study which found that, on average, women who ate yogurt regularly had a third the number of yeast infections as women who didn't. But be sure to buy yogurt that contains live cultures of *Lactobacillus acidophilus* or it won't be helpful. Or, instead, take acidophilus pills available in health food stores and some pharmacies.

• *Douche with a vinegar solution.* To help acidify your vagina, douche with a prepared vinegar solution or one of your own concoction (1 tablespoon vinegar to 1 quart of water).

Helpful Hints for Chronic Sufferers

Here are some tips to help prevent a yeast infection:

• Don't overindulge in sugary foods.
• Wear cotton panties or pants with cotton crotches.
• Do not wear skin-tight pants, tights, or panty hose if you are especially susceptible to yeast.
• Use sanitary pads instead of tampons. Never use tampons for a discharge or spotting but only for heavy flow.
• Eat at least a few ounces of live-culture yogurt a day.

- Never douche with anything but a vinegar solution.
- Don't hang about in a wet bathing suit for long periods of time.

TRICHOMONIASIS

A tiny protozoa, a distant relative of the amoeba, causes this variety of vaginitis that is, in truth, a sexually transmitted disease (STD) because it is usually passed along through intercourse. On the other hand, trichomonads may also live in moist warm environments such as wet towels and swimsuits and can be transmitted very easily.

Responsible for about 10 percent of all vaginal infections, *Trichomonas vaginalis* makes its presence known by a profuse vaginal discharge that is a frothy grayish or yellow-green, usually with a powerful and offensive odor. Not only that, but the organism causes burning, itching, and irritation of both the vulva and vagina. Sometimes there's spotting and almost always discomfort or even pain during sexual intercourse.

Men get trichomoniasis, too—and certainly pass it on—but fewer than one in five has symptoms. For men, it is often self-resolving; for women, it may last forever if it isn't treated.

The treatment is Flagyl (metronidazole) taken either in a single large dose or in smaller doses three times a day for a week. Your partner(s) must be treated at the same time if you don't want to get trichomoniasis right back again after you are cured. Don't drink alcohol while you're taking this medication or you may have some unpleasant side effects. Because this infection can be transmitted sexually, make sure you or your partner wears a condom.

BACTERIAL VAGINOSIS

Bacterial vaginosis (BV) is a new name for an old condition that used to be called "nonspecific vaginitis." The most prevalent of all vaginal infections, it is caused by an overgrowth of normal anaerobic bacteria, including the gardnerella organism, that results in 100 to 1,000 times more bacteria than are normally present in the vagina. Although any woman can get BV, sexually active women are most likely to get it. Men are susceptible also and, if you suffer with recurrent bouts, your partner should be treated, too.

Major symptoms are a milky discharge with an unpleasant, sometimes fishy, odor. Like other infections, it can cause itching or burning of both the vagina and the vulva, becoming very annoying if it's not treated quickly.

Once yeast infections and trichomoniasis are ruled out, a diagnosis of BV can be made quite easily by measuring the acid balance of the vagina or examining the cells under a microscope. The vagina will be much less acid than usual and the offending bacteria may be seen clinging to the vaginal cell walls.

The standard treatment method for BV is 5 grams (one applicator) of the antibiotic metronidazole vaginal gel (MetroGel) inserted into the vagina twice a day for five days; or 5 grams of clindamycin phosphate vaginal cream (Cleocin) inserted once a day for seven days.

VULVAR PAIN

A problem that few women—and even few physicians—know much about but others know only too well is *vulvodynia*, sometimes called *vulvar vestibulitis*. This is persistent stabbing and burning pain in the vulva, the external genital tissue that surrounds the opening of the vagina. It sometimes becomes so intensely painful, tender, itchy, stinging, swollen, and inflamed that some women can't even wear underwear and are uncomfortable sitting or walking. For many, the condition makes sexual intercourse unbearable and even walking an ordeal.

Until recently, no one knew what might cause vulvodynia. It tends to accompany interstitial cystitis (see page 310) and has been blamed on human papilloma virus, herpes, excessive levels of calcium oxalate in the urine, frigidity, vitamin deficiencies, and a vivid imagination. Recent research has brought relief to some women with supplements of calcium citrate and a diet very low in calcium oxalate. Other therapies include hormone creams, surgery, biofeedback, interferon, and low doses of tricyclic antidepressants.

For help and information, contact:

The Vulvar Pain Foundation
433 Ward Street
Graham, North Carolina 27253
919-226-0704

Chapter 12

YOUR CERVIX: HOW TO KEEP IT IN GOOD CONDITION

A WOMAN WHO HAS REGULAR PAP SMEARS never has to worry about developing cervical cancer. This is one disease that is 100 percent avoidable. Cervical cancer always begins as a precancerous condition called *dysplasia* (recently renamed cervical interepithelial neoplasia, or CIN for short) that develops into a malignancy only when it is neglected. Even when it has been allowed to turn into cancer, it is always curable if it is caught before it has spread beyond the surface layer of cells.

Luckily, dysplasia usually takes many years to turn into cancer, but that doesn't mean you are ever safe in ignoring it. It only means there's no need to panic if you get a report from your doctor of an abnormal Pap test.

We do see and treat many cases of dysplasia and occasionally even carcinoma in situ, but we rarely see cases of cervical cancer itself today. When we do, it is only in women who have not been regularly screened. Most of them, by the way, are older women who thought they needn't worry about their cervix at their age. Unfortunately, they are the ones who must be the most vigilant because the incidence of cervical cancer increases with age, and most cases are diagnosed in women who are between 40 and 60.

Despite a 70 percent decrease in cervical cancer deaths since Dr. George Papanicolaou invented the Pap smear early in this century, over 4,000 American women die each year from this kind of cancer. More than half of them have never had a single Pap smear and the rest haven't been screened frequently enough.

WHAT YOU CAN DO *NOW*

Schedule a Pap smear now and once a year hereafter (more often if you have recently had abnormal results). This quick screening test—a proven lifesaver that is still the only reliable early-detection technique for any kind of cancer—can pinpoint the future possible development of a malignancy up to ten years before it actually happens. Sounding an alarm at the first appearance of atypical cells, it allows for very early treatment and promises that a woman who has regular Pap smears never has to worry about getting cervical cancer. While no test is perfect, there's no screening method that is more effective than the Pap smear.

"Are there other ways to help yourself avoid dysplasia and/ or cervical cancer?"

A few. One, limit the number of sexual partners you have. The more partners, the more likely you are to get the human papilloma virus (HPV), the only known cause of cervical cell damage. Two, practice safe sex with new partners. Three, don't smoke. Cigarette smoking has emerged as a powerful influence in the development of both abnormal cervical cells and cancer of the cervix. In a recent study of women with advanced cancer at the Montefiore Medical Center in New York City, 85 percent were found to be smokers. And the remainder had had significant exposure to passive smoking.

Other evidence of the dangers of smoking turned up in a Norwegian study, which found that smokers are 50 percent more likely than nonsmokers to have cervical dysplasia, the risk rising with the numbers of cigarettes smoked per day and the years devoted to it. Whether nicotine acts as a carcinogen or smoking impairs the immune system is not known, but the fact that it encourages this kind of cancer as well as many others is a good reason to quit.

Helpful Hint

If you schedule a Pap smear *and* your yearly mammogram during the same month as your birthday, you'll be less likely to forget about it.

"I've never been sure exactly what the cervix is. Is it part of the vagina?"

No, it is part of the uterus, the narrowing lower portion that opens into the vagina. However, it consists of squamous tissue much like skin while the rest of uterus is made up of muscle and glandular tissue.

"What is a Pap smear?"

It is a sample of cells from the cervix, the endocervix (the transitional area between uterus and cervix), and the upper vagina. The sample is scraped or brushed in and around the cervix, smeared and fixed on a glass slide, and sent to a laboratory for microscopic examination by a trained technician called a cytotechnologist. At the lab, the cells are stained to make the details of the cells show up clearly under the microscope. Irregularities in the size and shape of the cells and their nuclei are reported back to the doctor as normal or abnormal.

"What does getting a 'positive' or 'negative' reading on a Pap test mean?"

A positive result means that atypical cells (cells of abnormal size or shape or dysplasia) have been found in the sample. If none are found, the Pap report is classified as negative or normal. Each year, about 10 percent of those tested are notified that their Pap test is abnormal, often a frightening announcement to women who don't know what it means. A positive Pap smear does not indicate that you have cancer or even a precancerous condition, but merely that investigation is needed. The Pap is a screening test and, in addition to dysplasia, it can detect yeast, trichamonas organisms, and gardnerella bacteria, as well as herpes and chlamydia.

"Can I trust the results of a Pap smear? What if it's been read wrong?"

The Pap smear is not and never has been 100 percent accurate, and that's why you should have one every year without fail. It is a screening test that is designed to alert your physician to disease in a cervix that looks perfectly normal. Even if it isn't read correctly one year, you'll get a second chance next year, with time enough for appropriate action.

Any *one* Pap smear has a 20 percent—or one in five—chance of not detecting the abnormal cells. The chance that it will be missed twice in a row falls to 4 percent. And the chance that it will be missed three times in a row is only a little over 1 percent. So after three consecutive yearly smears, virtually all women with abnormal cells on their cervixes can be identified.

"Why are mistakes made?"

About half the time it can be blamed on the physician, who misses getting a good sample of the small area on the cervix that happens to have abnormal cells. This is easy to do because the irregular cells often cannot be seen by the naked eye or the view may be obscured by blood or contaminants.

The other half of the false negatives occurs because of human error in reading the slides. Since the big flap in 1987 concerning "shoddy" Pap smear readings, a new regulation limits the number of slides a cytotechnologist may read in a day, making mistakes less likely to happen because of overload. In addition, the standard reporting system used by the labs to describe Pap smear abnormalities has been simplified and clarified. And currently under development is an automated computer system for interpreting Pap smears that promises to eliminate mistakes altogether.

Preparing for a Pap Smear

Do not schedule a Pap smear during a menstrual period because the blood can skew the test results. The best time is seven to ten days after the first day of your last period. For the same reason, for two days before the exam, no sex, douching, tampons, vaginal contraceptives, suppositories, vaginal medications, or estrogen cream.

"Is dysplasia the only problem that might show up on a Pap smear? Aren't there any other reasons for an abnormal Pap?"

Yes, but the only real concern is dysplasia. Everything else is relatively minor or even insignificant. Probably the major reason for "abnormal" Pap smears among women over 50 is inflammatory change because of atrophic vaginitis (see Chapter 11). This is a noninfectious inflammation of the lining of the vagina and cervix, a common condition after menopause unless you are taking hormone replacement. A bacterial or fungal infection, too, may be discovered on a Pap. The test cannot be relied upon to detect ovarian or uterine cancer, however.

"I keep getting told that I have cervicitis showing up on my Pap smear. What can be done about it?"

Cervicitis—chronic inflammation of the cervix—can be caused by bacteria or viruses, but sometimes it is simply an intermediate step in the body's ongoing self-repair process after injury or irritation. Its usual symptoms are spotting and/ or discharge. Cervicitis usually heals by itself eventually, but if it is very bothersome, it can be treated with cryotherapy, a simple office procedure. The affected area is frozen and destroyed and soon replaces itself with healthy tissue.

"My doctor found a polyp on my cervix. I've never heard of such a thing before. What is it?"

A polyp is a reddish protruding overgrowth of cervical tissue that usually causes no symptoms except perhaps spotting. Almost always benign, polyps should be removed for close examination just in case they are premalignant.

"What causes dysplasia?"

After many years of research, the prime suspect has been identified as the human papilloma virus (HPV), also called the condyloma virus. Thirty percent of American women (and at least as many men) are infected by this virus, which also causes genital warts (condyloma). Although HPV is almost always transmitted by sexual intercourse, it's probably possible to pick it up from bath towels, tanning booths, hot tubs, shower soap, or even gynecologic instruments.

The problem is that HPV, very easy to acquire and almost impossible to get rid of, can be passed along by a single act of intercourse. Unfortunately, there's no reliable way to prevent it. Even practicing safe sex with new partners, although it certainly has much to recommend it, may not always help you avoid it.

Because HPV may not produce abnormalities in cervical tissue for years or even decades—and won't show up on Pap smears until it does—it's impossible to know exactly where, when, or how you became infected. So if you are in a monogamous relationship and your Pap smear suddenly shows evidence of HPV infection, don't assume you got it from your current partner or he from you. More likely one of you got it from an earlier partner, perhaps long forgotten. But wherever it comes from, once you've got this infection you've probably got it for life. Sometimes it seems to vanish but, like many other viruses, this one may lay dormant for many years only to pop up once again when your resistance is low.

"What's the relationship between HPV and abnormal Pap smears?"

A third of women with HPV have perfectly normal Pap smears, while two-thirds of those with abnormal Pap smears have evidence of HPV. It is not known whether the virus itself eventually causes abnormal cells or whether it must first interact with another cellular event—such as a mutation, another infection, or a change in the immune system—to be activated. Meanwhile, the main message is: If you have HPV, have regular Pap smears. The second is: Be sure new sexual partners wear condoms backed up by spermicide.

"Does a diagnosis of papilloma (HPV/condyloma) mean I'm going to get cervical cancer some day?"

Certainly not. Cervical cancer from any source including the human papilloma virus is 100 percent preventable. Papilloma causes dysplasia (abnormal cells), which is pre-pre-pre-cancer. Properly treated, the dysplasia won't become cancer. On the other hand, if you don't take care of it, it could. Papilloma has become a national epidemic, and every gynecologist is kept very busy dealing with it; see Chapter 8.

"I always thought cervical cancer came from herpes. Is there a connection?"

No, although for a long time herpes was implicated because many women were found to have both herpes and cervical dysplasia.

"Does HPV always cause genital warts?"

Only in about 10 percent of the cases. Although the warts are usually small and painless, often too tiny or hidden away to be easily spotted, they are sometimes quite tender.

"What are genital warts?"

Small pink or gray raised areas usually found on the vulva, labia, cervix, or entrance to the vagina. Sometimes they appear at the outside of the urethra or around the anus. Warts in the vagina can be quite uncomfortable, causing itching, discharge, soreness, or bleeding, especially after intercourse. In one recent study of 82 women with anogenital warts, over half experienced tenderness or pain in the affected area and 23 percent of the sexually active women experienced pain during intercourse.

"What's the treatment for HPV and its genital warts? My friend had a terrible time with it."

There is currently no known cure for HPV. However, the warts can be removed if they are bothersome, perhaps decreasing the chances of transmitting the disease to somebody else. They can be eradicated with chemicals, cryosurgery (freezing), electrocautery (wire burner), or laser vaporization. See Chapter 8 for more about HPV.

VITAMIN PROTECTIONS

Aside from trying to avoid the human papilloma virus by not sleeping with people who have it or practicing safe sex, your best bet is to get into the habit of consuming adequate quantities of two vitamins thought to be protective of the cervix.

The first is folic acid (one of the B vitamins), which seems to help protect cervical cells from invasion by HPV, according to scientists at the University of Alabama at Birmingham, who recommend consuming at least 400 micrograms of folic acid in a daily multivitamin supplement and/or several servings of vegetables a day. Foods rich in folic acid are lima beans, whole wheat, brewer's yeast, wheat germ, liver, and leafy green vegetables.

The other is vitamin A, which also may provide some protection for the epithelial cells of the cervix. It is best taken as beta-carotene (too much straight vitamin A may be toxic); be sure you get an adequate amount in your daily diet or by supplements.

ARE YOU A PRIME CANDIDATE FOR HPV AND DYSPLASIA?

Considering that about three-quarters of American women today start having sexual intercourse in their teens and that they may have several sexual partners in a lifetime, all sexually active women should consider themselves at high risk for an abnormal Pap smear. High-risk factors for HPV include:

- Having started to have sexual intercourse as a teen-ager.
- Having had more than three sexual partners.
- Having a partner who has had more than three sexual partners.
- Being a smoker.

WHEN YOUR PAP SMEAR IS ABNORMAL

If your smear indicates the presence of atypical cells (dysplasia), the doctor will probably recommend two additional procedures: colposcopic examination and biopsy. A *colposcope*, which looks like binoculars on wheels, magnifies the cervix and helps determine the location of the abnormal cells. After anesthetizing the cervix, the doctor takes tissue samples (biopsies) of any suspicious-looking tissue, removing a small area with tiny sharp scissors and sending it off to be carefully examined by a pathologist. If the atypical area is reasonably contained, it can be completely removed during the biopsy and follow-up Pap smears are all that's necessary to be sure all of the abnormal cells are gone.

For a more extensive area of damaged cells, the usual treatment is cryotherapy, which destroys the cells by freezing them with nitrous oxide gas. Another choice is vaporizing them with a laser beam. Again, follow-up smears are required to make sure the tissue has been completely eradicated. Neither of these procedures should be painful, although they may be uncomfortable.

When there are more extensive or serious abnormalities or the atypical cells seen in the smear can't be located by colposcopy, a larger area of the cervix must be biopsied. This is accomplished by a *cone biopsy*, a technique that removes a fairly sizable cone-shaped section of the cervix for diagnosis and, when the entire area of abnormal tissue is removed, serves as treatment as well. Cone biopsies come in three different varieties, but whatever excision method is used, you should have a negative Pap smear by the time the treatment is completed.

- A "cold knife" cone biopsy, a surgical procedure performed in the hospital under general anesthesia, removes the sample of cervical tissue with a surgical scalpel.
- A laser accomplishes the same purpose but uses a laser beam as the cutting tool. This procedure is done in the hospital under general anesthesia.
- The newest technique for making a cone biopsy is the LEEP (loop electrosurgical excision procedure). Performed in the physician's office with local anesthesia, LEEP uses an electrified wire loop to scoop out the suspicious area.

"What's the follow-up treatment?"

After the dysplasia has been removed, you'll be asked to come back for Pap tests at least twice a year until the physician is certain that abnormal cells are gone for good.

Breaking News: Retin-A

The prescription cream Retin-A now used for acne and wrinkles may have health benefits that are more than skin deep: reversing cervical dysplasia. In a recent study financed by the National Cancer Institute, dysplasia reverted to normal tissue in 43 percent of the cases of women applying Retin-A to their cervixes compared to 23 percent of those using a placebo cream. The medication contains a synthetic variation of Vitamin A.

"And if it's cancer?"

A carcinoma in situ—cancer that is "in place" and has not yet invaded the surrounding tissue—can be removed by the same methods discussed above. An invasive cancer usually means that the whole uterus including the cervix must come out in a hysterectomy, followed up by Pap smears every four months for two years, then twice a year, then only once.

"If your cervix—and the rest of your uterus—has been removed by hysterectomy, must you continue to take Pap tests? What if you've had cervical cancer?"

If you have had cervical cancer, the most common place for a recurrence is in the part of the vagina that meets the cervix. It may be, in fact, an extension of the original cancer. Vaginal cancer is very rare, but we always watch for it by using the Pap smear, which will pick up abnormal vaginal cells before they turn into cancer. Besides, it is such a cheap and easy test that it makes no sense not to have one every year.

If you no longer have a uterus although you did not have cervical cancer, you should also continue to have Pap tests anyway. They are excellent indicators of vaginal health because they can detect bacterial and viral vaginal infections, provide an estimate of hormone levels, and rule out vaginal cancer.

Chapter 13

YOUR UTERUS: FIBROIDS, BLEEDING, AND OTHER HAPPENINGS

THE UTERUS, a hollow organ about the size and shape of an upside-down pear, is made up of an outer muscular layer called the *myometrium* and an inner glandular lining, the *endometrium*. The dome-shaped upper section of the uterus is the *fundus*, the central portion is the *corpus*, or body. The *cervix*, its best-known part, forms the base where the uterus narrows down to a small opening that meets the vagina. Because the cervix is composed of a different kind of tissue than the rest of this important organ and has a different set of problems, we have given it a chapter of its own (Chapter 12).

By the time you have reached the age of 40 or 50, you are not likely to spend much time thinking about your uterus—you're accustomed to your menstrual cycle and are probably not planning on adding a new member to the family—unless it calls itself to your attention. In this phase of your life that's usually accomplished by pain, discomfort, or bleeding at unscheduled times. And in most cases, your problem turns out to be fibroids.

FIBROIDS EXPLAINED

More than three-quarters of women over the age of 40 have or will develop fibroids (leiomyomas or myomas, for short)—nonmalignant tumors composed mostly of the same smooth muscle and fibrous connective tissue as the wall of the uterus. Some women have only one or two of these benign knots of tissue, but it's much more likely that they have developed clusters of them.

Fibroids may be as small as a grain of sand or as big as a basketball or even a full-term pregnancy. They are seldom painful and are not inherently dangerous, although they may cause abnormal bleeding, usually in the form of extra-heavy periods. But no matter how big they get, there is no reason to do anything about them if they don't cause significant problems.

Every fibroid begins with the mutation of a single uterine muscle cell resulting from an alteration in a gene or small group of genes that allows for deregulation of cell growth. The original mutated cell multiplies and, stimulated by estrogen, finally builds up into a firm whorled ball of tissue. Although fibroids are not initiated by estrogen, they depend on it for their growth, thriving best in the years when you produce plentiful hormones and shrinking after menopause when you don't.

Fibroids come in three varieties: intramural, submucous, and subserous. Intramural fibroids, the most common, grow within the walls of the uterus. Submucosal fibroids, growing under the uterine lining and into the uterine cavity, are the most likely to cause heavy bleeding. Subserous tumors form on the outer walls of the uterus, sometimes growing on their own little stalks. Whatever kind they are, these muscle tumors may cause significant symptoms but they are virtually always benign.

FAST FACTS ABOUT FIBROIDS

- One out of every seven women has a hysterectomy because of fibroids. One-third of all hysterectomies—almost 200,000 a year in the United States—is performed because of them.
- Black women are two or three times more likely to have fibroids than white women.
- Eighty-five percent of women with fibroids have many of them.
- Obese women have an increased risk of developing these benign tumors.
- Lean women who exercise regularly—and women who smoke cigarettes—have a lower risk of developing fibroids.
- Women who have had at least two full-term pregnancies and those who take low-dose oral contraceptives have a decreased risk for fibroids.
- Fibroids, which are estrogen-dependent, usually become large enough to start causing problems for women by the time they are in their late thirties or early forties, commonly growing fastest during the perimenopausal years, then shrinking after menopause.

"What causes fibroids?"

No one knows, but we do know they are usually genetically determined. In other words, if your mother had them, you are likely to have them too.

"What are the usual symptoms of fibroids?"

The most common significant symptoms are bleeding, feeling of pressure, and pain. Some fibroids cause extra-heavy menstrual bleeding or unscheduled irregular bleeding between periods. The bleeding, by the way, comes from the endometrium, the uterine lining, and not from the fibroids, which merely precipitate this response. However, these benign tumors can sometimes make the endometrium bleed so profusely that it causes serious anemia.

Other fibroids may become so large that they crowd the bladder or the bowel, producing a feeling of fullness and pressure that can be debilitating and even painful. When they sit on top of the bladder, they can cause bladder problems such as incontinence or urgency. And when they impinge on the rectum, they can cause constipation. Sometimes a large tumor will press against the stomach or diaphragm, resulting in gastric disturbances or shortness of breath. Or it can obstruct a ureter, one of the tubes leading from the kidneys to the bladder, encouraging kidney infections.

"How does the doctor know whether you have fibroids or something else?"

When your gynecologist feels an enlarged or irregularly shaped uterus during a pelvic examination—and has ruled out the possibility of pregnancy—it can quite safely be assumed that you have fibroids. If you have irregular bleeding, the small possibility of cancer is excluded by taking a sample of the uterine lining by endometrial biopsy or D & C. Then, if the diagnosis of fibroids is still in question, it may be verified in one of these ways:

- *Hysteroscopy.* The uterine cavity is illuminated and examined for the presence of fibroids or other problems through a hysteroscope, a small hollow tube fitted with a light and a magnifying lens, inserted vaginally into the uterus. This is an office procedure performed with local anesthesia.

- *Ultrasonography.* High-frequency sound waves are used to display the shape and density of the uterus on a TV screen. Ultrasound is painless and harmless, but it may not provide an absolutely certain diagnosis of fibroids.
- *Hysterosalpingogram.* In this ten-minute office procedure, X-ray pictures are taken of the uterus after it has been filled with a special liquid, allowing the outline of the irregular contours of the fibroids to be visualized if they are of the submucosal variety and protrude into the uterine cavity.

"Can fibroids be cured?"

The only sure cure is to remove them surgically, by hysterectomy or myomectomy. Sometimes, however, if you are in your late forties, fibroids will stop growing or even shrink enough to be tolerated until menopause, when your estrogen production will diminish dramatically.

"Are there other valid reasons besides severe pain, uncomfortable pressure, or heavy bleeding to remove fibroids?"

No. In the past it was felt that when fibroids grew to be greater in size than a twelve-week pregnancy, they were likely to cause symptoms and should therefore be removed. Besides, they could obscure the ovaries, making it impossible to examine them accurately for ovarian cancer or cysts during a pelvic exam.

The thinking today is that, as long as you are symptom-free, there is no need to take the fibroids out because, even when the ovaries can't be felt in the traditional pelvic exam, they can be visualized with ultrasound.

"I have a fibroid that's become very large very quickly. My doctor says it is not a problem but I worry that it could be cancer."

A rapidly growing fibroid used to be considered ominous, but today we know it's no more likely to become malignant than one that grows more slowly.

The Best Advice

Just because you have fibroids doesn't mean something must be done about them or that you are destined for surgery. The majority of women have no symptoms and never even know they have these tumors until their gynecologist detects them during a pelvic examination. The risk of cancer is very low, even for those that grow rapidly. Fibroids that are benign must be treated only if the problems they cause—bleeding, pain, pressure— become more than you care to live with.

DEALING WITH FIBROIDS SURGICALLY

When fibroids cause more trouble than you wish to put up with, a hysterectomy may well be the answer. But it is not always the only way to go. Today there are a few alternatives that have become increasingly popular. These include hormonal drugs that make fibroids shrink and surgical techniques that remove only the tumors, leaving the uterus intact.

Hysterectomy, or surgical removal—through the abdomen or the vagina—of the uterus, usually including the cervix, puts an end to fibroids once and for all. See page 282 for details.

Myomectomy is also an operation, but in this case only the tumors are removed and the uterus is left in place. Although myomectomies have been welcomed by many women who want to hold on to their uteruses—especially if they may want to become pregnant—it, too, usually involves major abdominal surgery. Each fibroid tumor is cut from the walls of the uterus and the uterus is sutured back together again. Sometimes, however, the fibroids can be removed by less invasive techniques (see below).

The main disadvantage of a myomectomy is that it doesn't guarantee that a new crop of fibroids won't develop again, although the chances decline with age. If they do grow again, they may require another operation or even a hysterectomy, which is why most gynecologists prefer the more radical operation for women past their childbearing days. Statistics show that one out of six women who have had a myomectomy has a subsequent hysterectomy because her fibroids have made a repeat appearance.

An alternative to an abdominal myomectomy is the removal of the tumors with the aid of a viewing device called a laparoscope. The laparoscope, a long thin tube with a light source and a lens system, is inserted through a tiny incision in the belly button while instruments are inserted through another small incision. The navel is the chosen site because its skin is thin and there is no heavy muscle tissue beneath it. The fibroids are then vaporized by laser or excised surgically and removed through the same incision. The procedure usually requires only a one-night stay in the hospital.

A third alternative is *hysteroscopic myomectomy,* which is appropriate only for small submucosal fibroids on the inner wall of the uterus that protrude into the uterine cavity. A hysteroscope, a hollow tube with a light and a lens system, is inserted vaginally. Then the fibroids are removed by scooping them out with an electrified wire loop, vaporizing them with a laser, or simply cutting or clamping them off. Performed in an operating room under general anesthesia, this procedure requires no abdominal incision or overnight hospital stay.

DEALING WITH FIBROIDS MEDICALLY

Some medications can be used to produce a temporary decline in estrogen production, encouraging large and troublesome fibroid tumors to shrink. The most effective of them is GnRH (gonadotrophin-releasing hormone), although it is seldom considered the final solution and is almost always used merely to buy time.

Here's how it works: A synthetic derivative of GnRH, a hormone released from a part of the brain called the hypothalamus, is taken by monthly injection or twice-daily nasal spray to stop the ovaries from making estrogen. This induces a temporary menopause, complete with hot flashes and night sweats. No longer fueled by estrogen, the fibroids shrink considerably within two or three months.

The major drawback of GnRH treatment is that the drug can be taken for only a few months at a time and its effects don't last. After you quit taking it, the fibroids start to grow again and may eventually become as much of a problem as they were before.

But in the meantime, their smaller size can make a hysterectomy or myomectomy easier and safer. If they shrink enough, the treatment may also allow for a vaginal hysterectomy rather than abdominal surgery or even removal of the fibroids alone through laparoscopic or hysteroscopic myomectomy.

For women in their late forties or early fifties who are very close to menopause, this synthetic hormone may control the growth of fibroids and prevent surgery altogether by creating menopause artificially until it happens on its own. Another strategy is to begin taking low-dose birth-control pills after GnRH treatment. Usually slowing the growth of the fibroids, they may continue to be used until menopause. Meanwhile, they reverse the uncomfortable menopausal symptoms triggered by the GnRH.

"I've just had menopause and don't want to take hormone replacement therapy because I am trying to get a very large

fibroid to shrink enough to avoid a hysterectomy. My problem is that I have a strong family history of osteoporosis. Any suggestions?"

Only rarely does HRT make fibroids grow because the estrogen dose is so small, but you may be the exception. If so, you could try taking calcitonin instead of HRT to protect your bones (see Chapter 4). Or, after having bone-density tests to make sure you are not at great risk for osteoporosis at the moment, you could simply wait a couple of years for the fibroids to shrink before starting hormone therapy. You have about three years of leeway before the most rapid postmenopausal bone loss begins.

But with your family history, you must do *something* to help yourself eventually or you may well end up with a broken hip or a few fractured vertebrae.

"Is there any way to prevent fibroids? My mother had a lot of trouble with them."

Not that anybody knows. You might try using low-dose birth-control pills as your contraceptive. Unlike the higher-dose pills of the past, they may slow down the growth of fibroids you already have.

ABNORMAL BLEEDING

Vaginal bleeding that's not according to plan requires prompt investigation, although in most cases it turns out to be nothing to get excited about. Usually it is caused by fibroids, polyps in the cervix or uterus, a hormonal imbalance, or perimenopause. But once in a while it is the symptom of a significant problem that must not be ignored, such as overproliferation of the uterine lining (hyperplasia) or even cancer. Or maybe it means you're pregnant. Vaginal bleeding, by the way, always comes from the uterus, *not* the vagina, although it comes *out* of the vagina.

Don't try to diagnose the problem yourself and don't decide to wait it out. Always consider unplanned bleeding to be abnormal until proven otherwise. Make an appointment with your gynecologist immediately for a thorough examination. Do it if you have always had regular periods but now skip periods, get extra periods, have periods that are extra heavy, or start spotting or bleeding at odd times.

In midlife, the reason will almost invariably turn out to be fibroids or perimenopause, but don't make that assumption on your own. And don't let your doctor make it either without investigation. Unscheduled bleeding is like a small-craft warning—it means there may be rough seas ahead. Check it out.

If you have already had menopause, the only bleeding that's allowed to occur without investigation is the light monthly period that may be induced by the progesterone when you are on hormone replacement therapy. Consider all other bleeding, even minor spotting, to be suspect.

ABNORMAL BLEEDING *BEFORE* MENOPAUSE

There are three major causes of abnormal vaginal bleeding in the years before menopause. In other words, while you are still menstruating, capable of reproduction, and producing a normal or only slightly decreased supply of estrogen.

Early Pregnancy Getting pregnant may be the last thing on your mind, but unless you've been using an effective contraceptive, spotting could mean just that. Although by the time you are 40-something, it is not as easy as it may once have been for you to get pregnant (see Chapter 10), it happens. And it is rarely planned. About 80 percent of the pregnancies of women in their forties are accidental.

Spotting—minor bleeding—is fairly common in early pregnancy and usually resolves after a few days with a perfectly normal pregnancy. Or it may be the earliest sign that you will miscarry. Half of all pregnancies end in miscarriage by age 45. If you are going to lose the embryo, the bleeding will probably become heavier and you will have cramps. There's also the remote possibility of an ectopic (tubal) pregnancy, especially if the bleeding is accompanied by pain. If you have pain, see your doctor immediately. Don't be put off by a busy schedule—yours or the doctor's—because an ectopic pregnancy can be an emergency.

Don't depend on a home pregnancy test. It can be useful *only* if the results come out positive. Some home kits are not sensitive enough to detect an early pregnancy or one that is in trouble, and may give you an untrustworthy false negative result.

Hormonal Imbalance Regular periods are the most reliable clue to normal hormonal function. They mean you have menstrual cycles that always occur within twenty-five to thirty-six days of the last one, with variations of no more than a week, no skipped months, and a predictable pattern of menstrual symptoms such as bloating, breast tenderness, amount of menstrual flow, and intensity of cramping. When hormone production is out of kilter, for whatever reason, you may have no periods at all, erratic periods, daily spotting, or frighteningly heavy bleeding.

The usual reason, as you move along through your forties on your way to menopause, is perimenopause (see Chapter 2). That's because you are no longer regularly releasing eggs every month. Without ovulation to stimulate the production of progesterone, the female hormone that schedules the shedding of the uterine lining, your cycles usually become erratic and your bleeding irregular.

You may choose to live with periods that come and go, wax and wane, and that's what most women do. But if you find them unsettling, you can switch them back to a regular pattern by taking progesterone supplements or, sometimes even better, oral contraceptives.

Anatomic Abnormalities In relatively rare cases, abnormal bleeding may be caused by infections, inflammation, or a growth that's almost invariably benign.

- *Vulva and vagina.* Except as the result of direct trauma, accidental or sexual, the vulva and vagina seldom bleed. Even cancer is rare in these parts of your anatomy and then it almost always appears only in women in their sixties and seventies.
- *Cervix.* The cervix is rarely the cause of vaginal bleeding, although it may produce minor spotting, especially after intercourse, if you have cervicitis, a chronic inflammation that may show up as an abnormal Pap smear. Persistent cervicitis can be treated with cryotherapy.
- *Polyps.* Sometimes a small tag of tissue called a polyp grows on the cervix, perhaps protruding into the vagina, and tends to bleed, especially after intercourse. Almost never malignant, polyps may be removed easily and painlessly in your doctor's office. Polyps may also grow out of the uterine lining where they occasionally cause irregular bleeding.
- *Fibroids.* These benign uterine muscle tumors are the major instigators of heavy irregular bleeding.
- *Adenomyosis.* In this rather unusual condition, cells from the uterine lining grow into the walls of the uterus, swelling each month like the lining and causing painful periods with heavy bleeding or irregular bleeding at odd times.
- *Cancer.* The primary symptom of both cervical and uterine cancer is abnormal bleeding. See Chapter 12 for more about cervical malignancies. For uterine cancer, read on.
- *Unexplained bleeding.* Sometimes no cause can be found for continuously heavy bleeding. When all possibilities have been ruled out, a hysterectomy may finally be the only answer. But when a woman wants to keep her uterus despite the trouble it is giving her, another procedure may be tried. This is endometrial ablation, when the uterine lining is electrically coagulated and destroyed,

leaving the uterus in place. This puts an end to the bleeding but creates another problem: now that the endometrium is gone, it can't bleed and so it cannot issue its classic warning of possible malignancy in the future.

ABNORMAL BLEEDING *AFTER* MENOPAUSE

Once you are certifiably menopausal, menstrual periods are just a memory. Now you will never have them anymore *unless* you are on hormone replacement therapy with the progesterone taken cyclically for several days each month. Then you will probably have very light regular periods, at least for a year or two. These brief menstrual responses occur like clockwork just after you stop taking the progesterone pills each month. Their purpose is to clear out the uterine lining built up by the estrogen you are also replacing. They will be short (two to five days), unclotted, and light. They will vary by no more than one or two days, and only slightly in the amount of flow.

If *any* bleeding occurs at *any* time other than those few days, consider it abnormal and have it checked out immediately. If the bleeding lasts longer than its allotted time, if it doesn't occur on schedule, if it is very heavy, or if it contains clots, report these facts to your doctor. If you are not taking progesterone and you *ever* see blood, see your doctor without delay. In other words, *any* postmenopausal bleeding that does not occur according to plan must be investigated. (For more about postmenopausal bleeding, see Chapter 3.)

UTERINE PROLAPSE

As you age, especially if you have had a few children and difficult vaginal deliveries, the muscles and ligaments that support the uterus and other pelvic organs loosen up, allowing the uterus to sag, sometimes so much that it prolapses into or even through the vagina. At the same time and for the same reason, the bladder, the urethra, and the rectum may also drop lower in the pelvis.

A mild prolapse produces no annoying symptoms, but as the uterus falls lower it may cause strange heavy sensations in the vagina. And if it becomes really severe, a uterus can drop so far that it feels like something is falling out. It also may cause loss of urinary control.

WHAT YOU CAN DO *NOW*

You can prevent pelvic relaxation to some degree by doing Kegel exercises to strengthen the muscles of the pelvic floor. See page 320 for a full description of how to do them. Also stay reasonably thin because too much weight (and too many radical changes in weight) can increase the abdominal pressure on the uterus.

Or you can use a pessary—a rubber device much like a diaphragm that fits around the cervix to help prop up the sagging uterus and keep it from protruding into the vagina. Combined with topical estrogen and exercises to strengthen the pelvic floor, it is effective for many women. A pessary must be carefully fitted by your physician and then removed every month for a good cleansing. Some women find it more trouble than it's worth because it can interfere with sexual intercourse and frequently causes vaginal irritation that, in turn, sets you up for infections.

And, of course, there's surgery. As a last resort, the uterus can be propped back in place or removed via hysterectomy. In fact, approximately 15 percent of all hysterectomies are performed for this reason. At the same time, a fallen bladder or rectum can be repositioned and its supports tightened.

DYSMENORRHEA (PAINFUL MENSTRUAL PERIODS)

For most women in midlife, menstrual cramps are history. But there are some menstruating women in their forties and fifties who continue to suffer through at least a few miserable days every month. Others are surprised to find that they're suddenly having menstrual cramps again after years without them, and still others experience them now for the very first time in their lives.

Menstrual cramps, which are simply strong uterine contractions, are precipitated by a high blood level of prostaglandin, an endometrial hormone released just before the onset of a period. A powerful hormone, the same one that's responsible for contractions during labor, prostaglandin also causes the headaches, nausea, and diarrhea that also often accompany menstrual periods.

WHAT TO DO ABOUT CRAMPS

- *Pain killers.* Neither aspirin nor acetaminophen does a good job of relieving menstrual pain, so try the antiprostaglandin drugs: Motrin, Advil, Naprosyn, Ansaid, Ponstel, Anaprox, Toradol, and Nuprin. For eight out of ten women, they relieve the cramps significantly, especially if you start taking them *before* the pain begins. Unfortunately, they sometimes have side effects such as headaches, dizziness, and gastrointestinal upset. Always take them with food or a little milk.
- *Calcium.* Increase your calcium intake to at least 1,500 milligrams a day. In a recent study, high calcium was found to relieve menstrual pain significantly.

- *Heat.* Other measures that can help relieve cramps include heat applied to the lower abdomen and a soak in a hot bath.
- *Home remedies.* Many women find relief from menstrual cramps in herbal brews such as raspberry leaf tea; yoga exercises to relax tense muscles; massage; magnesium supplements; certain positions such as kneeling with your bottom in the air and your head and shoulders on the floor. And some women find that extra exercise the day before their period begins (but not after) subdues the cramps.
- *Oral contraceptives.* If you are still in the market for contraception, you might try using low-dose oral contraceptives. They are not only highly reliable for preventing pregnancy but are also an effective treatment for monthly cramps.

A Caution on Cramps

If menstrual cramps are a new or a renewed phenomenon for you in your thirties or forties, make an appointment with your gynecologist for a pelvic exam. Their appearance at this time in your life suggests the possibility of fibroids, endometriosis, or adenomyosis.

ENDOMETRIOSIS

Endometriosis is a chronic disease that affects more than 5 million American women in their reproductive years, most of them in their thirties and forties. In severe cases, this strange condition with an astonishing variety of symptoms can be extremely painful, but nobody knows for sure what causes it or how to cure it.

Endometriosis occurs when tissues normally found in the endometrium migrate outside of the uterus, implanting in sites where they don't belong. They grow on and around other tissue, most often the ovaries, the fallopian tubes, and the ligaments supporting the uterus. But sometimes they grow on the bladder, bowel, intestines, the outside of uterus, the interior walls of the pelvic cavity, in old surgery scars, or anywhere else in the abdomen and sometimes out of it. In some rare cases, endometriosis has even been found in such remote locations as the lungs. Most of the time, the deposits of endometrial tissue grow in tiny areas of inflammation. But on the ovaries they can form into spheres of clotted blood called endometriomas, sometimes as large as a grapefruit.

Endometriosis behaves just like the glandular lining of the uterus, responding to the monthly hormonal fluctuations of the menstrual cycle. Even though they are in some abnormal site, endometrial cells swell, break down, and shed each month. But unlike normal menstruation, there's no mechanism for evacuating this tissue at the end of every cycle. So it stays put, slowly increasing in size and causing irritation, inflammation, and scar tissue. The scar tissue can turn into fibrous adhesions that can eventually bind pelvic contents together, become excruciatingly painful, and cause infertility and problems with bowel and bladder function. Luckily, endometriosis rarely becomes malignant and, because it is estrogen-dependent, subsides after menopause.

The symptoms of endometriosis are painful—sometimes incapacitating—periods, pain or bleeding with urination or bowel movements, irregular bleeding or spotting between periods, painful sex, painful bowel movements, and infertility. Not so commonly, endometriosis may also cause lower back pain, intestinal upset, even shortness of breath, sciatica, and more. Because of its wide variety of symptoms, it has been called "the great masquerader."

One of the puzzles of this disease is that the severity of symptoms is not necessarily related to the severity of the condition. Women who have extensive endometriosis sometimes have no symptoms at all, while those who have only two or three small misplaced implants may have excruciating pain every month and find intercourse unbearable.

Certainly menstrual cramps (especially when you are many years beyond adolescence), painful intercourse, and pelvic pain should be enough to make you and your doctor suspect this strange disease. So should infertility. A third of the women with endometriosis are infertile—twice the rate in the general population.

Although this disease may be tentatively diagnosed by a simple vaginal examination or vaginal ultrasound, there are no accurate laboratory tests for it and a definitive diagnosis may be made only by laparoscopy. Laparoscopy is a minor surgical procedure done under anesthesia in which your abdomen is first stretched with carbon dioxide gas. A laparoscope (a tube with a light in it) is then inserted into a tiny incision in the belly button. This allows the surgeon to see and then evaluate the location, extent, and size of the implants.

There's no sure cure for endometriosis, but the current treatments are hormones that produce a temporary menopause, eliminating periods and swelling implants, for up to six months; surgical removal of the implants and scar tissue; or hysterectomy as a last resort. The decision about which way to go is influenced by your age, your future childbearing plans, the severity of the symptoms, and the location and extent of the scarring and inflammation.

For more information contact:

Endometriosis Association
8585 N. 76th Place
Milwaukee, Wisconsin 53223
800-992-ENDO

HORMONE THERAPY FOR ENDOMETRIOSIS

Hormone therapy is based on the observation that, although estrogen doesn't initiate the stray implants, it makes them grow. Treatment with hormones can suppress the disease, although it doesn't cure it, by preventing ovulation and the release of female hormones, forcing endometriosis into remission. Without nourishment, the misplaced tissue starts to shrink.

There are three disadvantages of hormonal treatment for endometriosis: they work only while you are taking them; they can cause significant side effects including all of the very worst menopausal symptoms; and the most effective drugs are very expensive.

Here are the choices:

1. *Combination oral contraceptives.* These are the least expensive hormonal treatment available. Taken daily, they inhibit the development of egg follicles, prevent ovulation, and stop menstruation. Safe, inexpensive, and convenient, they do have their side effects: breast tenderness, breakthrough bleeding, weight gain, and, in some women, depression.

2. *Danazol.* Marketed as Danocrine, this is a derivative of the male sex hormone testosterone, chemically modified

to eliminate most of the usual male side effects. It, too, disrupts the hormonal cycle and stops ovulation, suppressing estrogen production and menstruation. Usually prescribed for six months, it is taken in ever-decreasing doses. The possible side effects—which may include facial hair, fluid retention, dry vagina and other menopausal symptoms, fatigue, muscle cramps, headaches, and breakthrough bleeding—are usually mild and transient, vanishing when the treatment ends.

3. *GnRH agonists.* Synthetic derivatives of GnRH (gonadotrophin-releasing hormone), these induce a temporary menopause. Currently considered the most promising treatment although the most expensive, they block ovulation and stop menstruation, thereby causing the misplaced tissue to retreat. Taken by injection once a month (Lupron) or by nasal spray (Synarel) twice a day, GnRH treatment is usually prescribed for only six months at a time.

News Break

RU-486, the French-manufactured "abortion pill," which should be available in the United States in a year or two, may have potential use in the treatment of endometriosis as well as other common hormone-related female disorders, according to a recent report from the Institute of Medicine.

SURGICAL SOLUTIONS FOR ENDOMETRIOSIS

If you have very severe symptoms and all other therapy has failed, you will be faced with surgery as the only alternative, by itself or in combination with hormonal therapy. You must decide, with your doctor's help, whether you want to try a conservative approach or are willing to trade in your pain for extensive surgery or even a hysterectomy.

1. *Laparoscopic surgery.* With the guidance of a laparoscope, the extraneous implants are cut out, cauterized, or vaporized with laser through a small incision near the navel. In the same procedure, adhesions can be cut away, cysts drained, and damage repaired, leaving the uterus and usually one ovary and tube intact. The main advantage of the conservative approach is that it avoids major abdominal surgery and a big incision. The chief disadvantage is that the recurrence rate is high.

2. *Abdominal surgery.* When the implants are too large or extensive to remove through laparoscopic-assisted surgery, the migrant tissues must be taken out through a regular abdominal incision. This is obviously a more invasive procedure and means a longer recovery time.

3. *Hysterectomy.* The most radical surgery and the only definitive cure for endometriosis is a hysterectomy, with the ovaries removed as well. Only by completely removing the extensive implants and adhesions that have wrapped themselves around other tissue and, at the same time, shutting down the production of estrogen necessary for their growth, can the disease be effectively stopped. This, of course, induces instant menopause and everything that goes along with it.

   Abdominal hysterectomy is usually the only option because in most cases the entire abdomen must be exhaustively investigated. Besides, a vaginal hysterectomy is difficult and tricky when there are more than a few adhesions.

"If I have a hysterectomy and lose my ovaries because of endometriosis, should I take hormone replacement? Won't it make the tissue grow again?"

It would make your life much more pleasant if you do take HRT because it will eliminate the hot flashes, dry vagina, and other miserable menopausal symptoms that tend to be especially severe among women who have instant menopause. It will also decrease your long-term risk of osteoporosis and heart disease.

However, although HRT rarely stimulates the growth of more endometrial implants, you will have to be watched carefully because about 5 percent of women taking replacement hormones have a recurrence of the disease. And your dosage may have to be adjusted. You may do fine on the standard estrogen dose, but some women do better with a smaller dose that will do away with the menopausal symptoms but won't reactivate the endometriosis.

Some doctors recommend delaying the start of HRT for at least three months—and sometimes as long as nine months—after the surgery to allow any remaining implants to wither away, minimizing your chances of recurrence. If you do this, however, you will have to tough it out with the symptoms in the meantime, unless you take specially prescribed HRT that contains mainly or only progesterone.

"I've heard that getting pregnant will cure my endometriosis. Is that true? I'd be willing to have another baby if that would do it."

Sorry, but that's a myth. Almost invariably, pregnancy provides only a temporary interruption, giving relief from the symptoms while you are pregnant and perhaps a little longer.

ADENOMYOSIS

Adenomyosis is another condition that results in endometrial tissue migrating to a strange location, but this time the cells of the uterine lining invade only the muscular wall of the uterus, where they grow and respond to fluctuating hormone levels by swelling each month. Usually first diagnosed in women in their forties who have had children, adenomyosis causes extremely painful periods with heavy bleeding and sometimes irregular bleeding at other times of the month.

To date, there's no good treatment short of a hysterectomy for this disease and, in fact, a diagnosis is often made on the basis that all treatment has failed. In severe cases, the only relief from the pain comes when the enlarged uterus is removed. If you can live with the symptoms until menopause, however, you will find that the pain disappears on its own.

HYPERPLASIA AND ENDOMETRIAL CANCER

Endometrial cancer, like cervical cancer, is virtually 100 percent preventable. It goes through many stages on its way to becoming a malignancy and, if you go to your doctor regularly for complete gynecological examinations and between them if you have unscheduled vaginal bleeding, it can be picked up long before it ever gets there.

Uterine cancer almost invariably goes through a hyperplastic stage first. That means an abnormal proliferation of endometrial cells (the cells forming the uterine lining) so that it becomes thicker than it should be. This is not cancer, but it is a precancerous condition. Among the few women predisposed to endometrial cancer, hyperplasia can develop into a malignancy if it is neglected. On the other hand, not every case of hyperplasia turns into cancer even if it's left untreated.

A rare but more virulent form of endometrial cancer, unrelated to estrogen, is often diagnosed at a later stage and has a much poorer prognosis.

FAST FACTS ABOUT ENDOMETRIAL CANCER

- The incidence of confirmed cancer of the uterine lining is about 1 per 1,000 in a normal population.
- Most women who get it are past menopause and in their fifties, sixties, or seventies.
- The survival rate when it is caught before it has spread beyond the uterus is 92 percent.
- Your risk of developing endometrial cancer is doubled if your mother had it. The risk is also higher in women whose mothers have had breast cancer.
- A major trigger for endometrial cancer seems to be unopposed estrogen—in other words, estrogen without the protective effects of progesterone. This kind of cancer is rare before menopause except in women who never (or seldom) ovulate and so do not produce progesterone. After menopause, some women continue to make significant estrogen in their fatty tissue, building up the lining, but stop producing progesterone, which stimulates the shedding of that lining as a menstrual period. These women face higher risk.
- Taking estrogen replacement without taking progesterone along with it is another way of getting unopposed estrogen and increasing your risk of endometrial cancer. If you take estrogen and want to be absolutely safe, you must also take progesterone.
- Tamoxifen, the antiestrogen drug used to treat breast cancer and now under consideration for use in preventing breast cancer, may increase the chances of getting cancer of the uterus. Two studies of more than

5,000 women show that those taking tamoxifen face a risk of uterine cancer that is two to three times higher than that of the general population. The studies are continuing, but the early evidence was strong enough to prompt the FDA to issue warnings about tamoxifen's possible effects on the uterus. At the same time, the agency stated that the drug's benefits outweigh the risks.

• Your risk of developing hyperplasia and endometrial cancer is increased if you are diabetic, obese, or hypertensive.

Hyperplasia, luckily, warns you of its presence. It bleeds. It bleeds at unscheduled times or, if you haven't had menopause, it produces very heavy menstrual periods. If you go to your gynecologist whenever you have irregular, unexpected, or extra-heavy bleeding, you will be tested for hyperplasia with an endometrial biopsy, ultrasound, or, in some cases, a D & C (dilatation and curettage).

If the test indicates that the uterine lining is too thick, you will be treated with progesterone. With two or three months of progesterone, usually taken every day for a month and then for twelve days per month, the lining will almost always slough off its excessive buildup and return to normal. If that doesn't do the job, further investigation is essential.

TESTING YOUR ENDOMETRIUM

If there is any question that all is not well with your uterine lining, an exploration and examination are in order. Here are the usual procedures for determining its status:

Endometrial Biopsy or Aspiration: This is the retrieval of a small sample of tissue from the uterine lining and a microscopic examination of the cells by a trained pathologist. An office procedure that takes only a couple of minutes and occasionally causes minor cramping, it is usually done quite painlessly today with a pipelle. A slender catheter, the pipelle is inserted vaginally through the cervix and into the uterus, where it uses suction to remove a sample of endometrial tissue to be sent to a laboratory for testing.

Handy Hint

Take two antiprostiglandin tablets (Advil, Motrin, Anaprox, etc.) an hour or two before the procedure to minimize the possibility of cramping.

Dilatation and Curettage (D & C):   The D & C is a minor fifteen-minute operation usually performed in a hospital under general anesthesia. After the cervix is dilated, a spoon-shaped instrument called a curette is inserted into the uterus where it is used to scrape out the uterine lining. Samples of the tissue are sent to a laboratory for examination by a pathologist who looks for abnormal or excessive numbers of cells.

D & Cs have been almost totally replaced by endometrial biopsies or aspirations—procedures performed in the doctor's office. But when the uterus is very large, the bleeding very heavy, or the cervix too narrow to admit the pipelle, it is usually necessary. And in most cases, it is also the next step when too little tissue has been retrieved in the biopsy, when abnormal bleeding persists, or when abnormal cells have been detected in the tissue retrieved by biopsy.

Transvaginal Ultrasound: Used only for screening because it produces no cells for microscopic examination, ultrasound is used more and more frequently today to provide a valuable clue to the status of your uterus. It allows the physician a practical way to measure the thickness of the endometrium. If this lining has not overproliferated and therefore is thin, you are pronounced safe. If it is thick, it requires further investigation by biopsy.

Progesterone Challenge Test: An excellent way to test the endometrium and let you know if anything abnormal is going on, this can be a good screening test after menopause. If you don't bleed after taking 10 milligrams a day of oral progesterone for twelve days, it's most unlikely that you have hyperplasia. If you do bleed, indicating overproliferation of the lining, your doctor will then perform a biopsy to determine more precisely what's going on.

"Why can't a Pap test be used to detect hyperplasia or endometrial cancer?"

A Pap smear, designed to detect abnormalities of the cervix, is not a reliable test for abnormal uterine cells. That's because abnormal cells may not appear on the slide if they originate high in the uterus far from the cervix.

"What's the treatment for endometrial cancer?"

Surgery (a hysterectomy) or radiation, or a combination of the two.

"Why does being overweight increase the risk of endometrial cancer?"

Probably because the fat tissue converts certain hormones made by the adrenal glands into estrone, a form of estrogen, even after menopause. Estrone, unopposed by progesterone, can cause overproliferation of the uterine lining. The risk of endometrial cancer goes up about five times for women who are truly obese. Any woman who weighs much more than she should—certainly anyone who weighs over 200 pounds—is strongly advised to have a yearly biopsy or measurements via ultrasound to be sure she is safe. Being overweight and diabetic compounds the problem. If you are in that category, your risk goes up even more.

By the way, one recently reported study shows that women with this cancer have significantly greater amounts of fat in their upper bodies than healthy women do. So losing weight, especially for those with their fat concentrated above their waists, is a good way to reduce the risk.

"Why are diabetics more likely to get it?"

Nobody knows why diabetics have an increased risk for this cancer, but it is known that they tend to have abnormally high levels of circulating estrogen.

"Are you more susceptible to endometrial cancer if you have high blood pressure?"

Yes, perhaps because many hypertensives are also obese and/ or diabetic.

"I really need estrogen replacement because I have a family history of osteoporosis and heart disease, but I can't seem to tolerate progesterone. Is there any way to get along without it?"

Only if you are followed closely and, if necessary, treated for hyperplasia. We now consider it sufficient to measure the thickness of the endometrium with ultrasound (a thin lining is what we look for) once a year if you are not experiencing any kind of suspicious bleeding. But if there is bleeding or any other reason to suspect trouble, you must have periodic endometrial biopsies. Better to take progesterone (try a different form or brand) if you can manage to live with its side effects.

HYSTERECTOMY: ALMOST ALWAYS A JUDGMENT CALL

No woman is delighted to be told she needs a hysterectomy, yet one out of every three women in the United States has one before she reaches the age of 60. More and more, the need for this operation is being questioned by both medical experts and women's advocacy groups, especially when perfectly healthy ovaries are removed at the same time.

It is certainly true that far too many hysterectomies are routinely performed on women who don't understand the emotional and physical consequences of the procedure or who haven't been thoroughly informed about their options—one of which may be to do nothing at all. Hysterectomy is a major operation, and complications can and do occur. In addition, many women feel defeminized by the loss of their uterus even when their ovaries are left inside their bodies where they belong.

On the other hand, there are often valid medical reasons for removing a problem uterus when its symptoms have become too troublesome to live with.

Deciding whether the benefits of a hysterectomy will compensate for the trauma and the effects of the procedure, especially if you are still in your childbearing years, is almost always a pure judgment call. Except in cases of cancer, or for bleeding so heavy that a large amount of blood is lost very quickly, hysterectomy is never an absolute necessity. And watching and waiting is often the appropriate response for conditions that are not life-threatening, with treatment almost always depending on how unbearable the symptoms become.

So most of the time, quality of life is the major factor in the decision about whether or not to have a hysterectomy. Will you be better off with or without your uterus? Your ovaries? Are there valid alternatives? Should they be tried first? Is a hysterectomy too high a price to pay for the results you can expect to get? Can conservative treatments solve the problem and are you willing to take a chance that they will? These are decisions that should be made by *you* in consultation with your doctor, with a second or even a third opinion if you have any reason to question the need for this procedure. A recent study has found that hysterectomies are less likely to be performed when women question their doctor's recommendation. It also found that younger gynecologists chose this option less frequently.

FAST FACTS ABOUT HYSTERECTOMIES

- Hysterectomy, strictly speaking, is the surgical removal of the uterus including the cervix (or a portion of it). But almost a third of the time, especially among women over 40, both a hysterectomy and an oophorectomy—removal of the ovaries and fallopian tubes—are performed during the same procedure.
- Hysterectomies are second only to cesarean sections as the most common major operation in the United States. About 600,000 of them are performed a year, two-thirds on women under the age of 45. More than one out of every three women in the country over the age of 60 has had one.
- Women in the United States have more hysterectomies than in any other Western country, nearly six times as many as in Norway, Sweden, or England.
- A third of all hysterectomies are performed because of large troublesome fibroids—those benign muscular uterine tumors that may cause heavy bleeding and other problems. Other generally accepted reasons for a hysterectomy include excessive bleeding and anemia, uterine prolapse, pressure on other organs, endometriosis, and, of course, uterine cancer.

- The peak age for hysterectomy is 45.
- Recent research finds that hysterectomy slightly reduces the risk of ovarian cancer.

HYSTERECTOMY—WHAT IS IT?

Hysterectomy is major surgery that requires several weeks, perhaps several months, of recuperation. The downside includes possible infections, blood loss resulting in a 10 percent chance of transfusions, a one-in-a-thousand chance of dying from complications, and injury to the intestines or urinary tract—pretty much the same as for any other major abdominal surgery.

Abdominal hysterectomy, the most common technique, is the removal of the uterus through an incision made in the abdominal wall. This route must be taken when you have very large fibroids, when there is a suspicion of cancer, when a good look at your ovaries or other internal organs is required, or when, because of previous surgery or infection, the uterus is enveloped by scar tissue.

If you have a choice, request the low horizontal "bikini" incision, made just below the pubic hair line. It will be stronger and less visible, and will heal with less pain. If a larger view and more working space are needed, however, you will have to settle for a more noticeable vertical incision down the middle.

In a *vaginal hysterectomy*, the uterus (usually including the cervix) is removed through the vagina with no abdominal incision and therefore no scars. It is usually faster than an abdominal procedure, requires less anesthesia, and results in a shorter hospital stay, less pain, fewer complications, and a quicker recovery time. On the other hand, it is used only in less complicated cases because it does not allow for a thorough examination of the abdominal cavity and it won't work with very large fibroids. In addition, it is a more difficult operation, requiring more skill and experience on the part of the physician.

An increasingly popular technique, the *laparoscopically assisted vaginal hysterectomy* is the newest version of this procedure, although it is not always the best choice because it can take many hours to perform. A tiny incision is made in the abdominal wall through which a laparoscope, akin to a small lighted telescope at the end of a long thin tube, is inserted into the pelvic cavity where it provides a close-up view of the contents. Guided by an external video monitor, specially designed miniature instruments are then inserted through another small incision, and used to clamp off blood vessels and detach the uterus from its supports. The uterus is then "delivered" through the vagina.

By the way, prospective abdominal surgery can sometimes be converted to the vaginal variety by taking a GnRH agonist (see page 273) for about three months before the operation. The purpose is to shrink very large fibroids down to a more manageable size.

SHOULD YOUR OVARIES COME OUT TOO?

If you are scheduled for a hysterectomy and are over 40 to 45, it will probably be suggested that your ovaries be removed at the same time. Arguments rage on about the wisdom of taking out healthy ovaries, a practice that has become extremely controversial.

The argument *for* routinely removing them is that you are either fast approaching menopause or have already passed it. You're not going to need your ovaries anymore because your childbearing days are almost or totally over, so it makes sense to eliminate the possibility of future ovarian cancer, a deadly disease with no early warning signs.

The argument *against* removing healthy ovaries is that the risk of ovarian cancer is very small, less than 2 percent. This risk must be measured against the dramatic effects of losing all of your ovarian function. For some women, the loss of their reproductive organs is viewed as castration and defeminization. For all women who are still menstruating, it produces instant menopause. From that moment on, they will make no more estrogen (except for the small amount produced by the fat tissue).

Because your hormone supply has been so abruptly ended, you will probably suffer from the most severe menopausal symptoms, starting within a day or two after the surgery. In fact, the younger you are at the time of the surgery, the worse the symptoms are likely to be and the longer they will tend to last (unless, of course, you start hormone replacement therapy immediately after the operation).

Another risk of an early menopause is extra years without the protection estrogen gives your bones and your heart, and more years spent living with the atrophic effects of an estrogen-deficient vagina.

If you have already had menopause, losing your ovaries isn't so dramatic, but it does mean you will no longer have the benefits of the remnants of estrogen you may still produce. And you will lose the effects of other hormones that the ovaries continue to secrete. These are the malelike hormones—the androgens—that are responsible for libido in both men and women.

Occasionally a compromise is made. Only one ovary is removed, theoretically cutting down the risk of ovarian cancer (by much less than half, however) while allowing the remaining ovary to continue doing its job.

The decision about losing or keeping your healthy ovaries should be yours to make—with guidance, of course. Be sure you know what your doctor plans to do, make sure you understand and agree with the reasoning, and discuss your options.

By the way, even when you keep your ovaries, the hysterectomy may put you out of the estrogen business years ahead of schedule. Probably because the blood supply to the pelvic region is compromised, menopause may arrive much earlier than expected.

"I had a hysterectomy last year. Should I still have regular pelvic exams and Pap smears?"

Yes. If you still have your ovaries, it's important for your gynecologist to check them and your fallopian tubes periodically. And even if you haven't, you should have a vaginal checkup and a breast exam at least once a year. The Pap smear is still necessary, too, because the cells at the upper end of the vagina are similar to those of the cervix (which has been removed along with the rest of your uterus) and can become abnormal.

"I've been told that having a hysterectomy could ruin my sex life. Is there any truth in that?"

Although this is a subject of great concern to many women, most physicians believe that simple hysterectomies do not affect sexuality except perhaps psychologically. In our own personal experience, we have never seen sexual problems except among a few women who have felt they have lost their femininity along with their uterus.

But it's quite another story if your ovaries are also removed. Not only will you lose your major supply of estrogen, but you will lose your supply of androgens, the male hormones that are also almost totally produced in the ovaries. Testosterone, one of the androgens, is thought to be responsible for the sex drive in both men and women, although women's sexual response is complicated by cultural and psychological expectations. Many women feel a real reduction in sexual response without their ovaries.

"What can be done about that?"

Testosterone in tiny doses can restore your interest in sex in very short order—*if* your diminished libido stems from a shortage of it. It can be taken alone or in combination with estrogen, thus solving all of your current hormone problems at once. See Chapter 7.

"Isn't the cervix important in sexual response? Won't I lose my interest in sex without it?"

It's most unlikely. Only in very unusual cases is there ever direct contact between the penis (average length of an erect penis is 6 centimeters) and cervix (average length of a vagina is 8 centimeters). Besides, studies have found that the cervix does not contract with orgasm.

Chapter 14

YOUR OVARIES: COPING WITH PROBLEMS

THE OVARIES ARE a pair of pearly, almond-shaped glands about the size of walnuts that are suspended below the fallopian tubes on either side of the uterus. Because they produce eggs and the female hormones estrogen and progesterone, their function is vital to your well-being as a woman. By the time you have reached 40 or 50, however, your only concerns about them have probably narrowed down to the possibility of cysts and your chances of developing ovarian cancer.

OVARIAN CYSTS

Once a month, every menstruating woman produces a benign ovarian cyst, a tiny encapsulated fluid-filled sac, on an ovarian follicle. As an egg matures inside it, it ruptures and releases the egg during ovulation. But if an egg fails to ovulate, the sac may continue to grow, forming a follicular cyst. Because it develops from normal tissue that changes with ovulation every month, it is called a functional cyst and usually disappears before the next menstrual period. If it doesn't, it must be watched and investigated.

Another physiological variety of cyst can develop in the small cavity created in the ovary after an egg has been expelled. This cavity fills in with blood vessels and new cells to form the corpus luteum, which then begins to secrete progesterone in preparation for pregnancy. Usually the corpus luteum lasts for two weeks, then, if there's no pregnancy, shrivels up to form a tiny scar. But if the ovarian surface bleeds into the corpus luteum, a cyst may form, filled in by the blood. This, too, usually disappears within a month or two.

Other common ovarian cysts are actually small tumors that become filled with fluid or even fat and hair (a dermoid cyst). Some fill up with mucus and have been known to grow as big as full-term pregnancies. And still others are caused by endometriosis (see Chapter 14).

Seven out of ten ovarian cysts are the functional variety and go away on their own by the next menstrual period. If a cyst persists longer, causes pain or bleeding, and/or grows very large, obviously it requires investigation. In most cases, a pelvic ultrasound examination will reveal its type, size, and chances of causing trouble or being malignant.

Most ovarian cysts are symptomless; you'd never know you had one if your doctor didn't feel it during a routine pelvic exam or spot it on ultrasound. But when they grow very large, they may press against your bladder or your rectum or the abdominal wall. Once in a great while, a cyst causes severe sudden pain, perhaps accompanied by nausea, when it ruptures or twists on itself. The pain usually disappears rather quickly but sometimes it persists. Either way, you must promptly check it out with your gynecologist.

WHAT YOU CAN DO *NOW*

Schedule a pelvic exam. If you haven't had a pelvic examination within the last year, schedule one now. Every woman needs regular routine checkups of her reproductive tract, no matter her age. Without a pelvic exam, you may not become aware of an ovarian cyst until it grows very large and causes symptoms.

Any cyst that doesn't disappear in a month or so and grows larger than about 5 centimeters in menstruating women and 2 centimeters in postmenopausal women requires a thorough investigation and, in most cases, must be removed even if it appears to be perfectly benign. That's to avoid the possibility of rupture or twisting and to make sure it is among the vast majority of cysts that are nonmalignant. A color ultrasound will help the doctor decide what variety it is and whether or not it looks suspicious.

A CA-125 blood test can also provide clues (see below), especially in women who are no longer menstruating. A postmenopausal woman with a benign ultrasound appearance and a normal CA-125 has very little chance of having a malignant cyst.

Cysts can be removed by laparoscopy (through small incisions near the belly button) except when they are large or the ultrasound results are in doubt. Then an abdominal operation—a laparotomy—is more likely to be the choice so the doctor can get a better view of your ovaries and your other reproductive organs.

"Why can't these cysts simply be drained rather than removed if they are harmless?"

Because they tend to recur after they have been aspirated. Besides, only their complete removal allows for the thorough examination under a microscope that can definitively confirm they are benign.

"Do you usually have a hysterectomy when you have ovarian cysts removed? That's what happened to my mother."

Not anymore, although time was when that was standard practice. Any woman beyond menopause with benign ovarian cysts was routinely treated to an abdominal operation that included a hysterectomy—removal of her uterus—in the name of preventing future problems. Today, however, the more conservative approach is the usual choice. According to a recent study, women who have a benign ovarian mass and a healthy uterus fare better without a hysterectomy.

"Am I more likely to get cancer because I have had benign ovarian cysts? If so, I'd like to have my ovaries removed."

The answer is no. You are not more susceptible to cancer simply because of cysts.

OVARIAN CANCER

Ovarian cancer is the fourth leading cause of cancer deaths in women, with about 22,000 new cases diagnosed every year in the United States. Rare in a woman under 40, its incidence increases every year after that, although it is not nearly as common as cancer of the lung, breast, or colon. It is easily cured in its earliest stage, but this cancer is a particularly nasty one because, while only one woman in seventy gets it, few cases are discovered early. Unlike cervical or endometrial cancers, which grow very slowly and can be detected in their premalignant stage, ovarian cancer invades the body silently and has usually spread to other parts of the body by the time it is diagnosed. Ovarian cancer is nefarious because it issues no early-warning signals: no bleeding, no pain, no lumps, no other symptoms or signs of trouble. Nor are there any ideal screening tools to help catch it in its early stages.

WHAT YOU CAN DO *NOW*

Have a yearly gynecological checkup, when your physician will examine your ovaries by feeling for irregularities and size. Let your doctor know if you have a strong family history of ovarian malignancies so that you can be watched more carefully and tested more frequently.

Ask your doctor about the wisdom of going on oral contraceptives. Often prescribed for women with family histories of this disease, they have been found to cut the risk of both ovarian and endometrial cancers by more than half. What's more, the protection lasts for at least fifteen years after you quit taking them.

When genetic testing for a defective gene that predisposes some women to ovarian cancer becomes available, ask to be screened if this cancer runs in your family.

For more information on ovarian cancer, call the Gilda Radner Familial Ovarian Cancer Registry, 800-682-7426.

FAST FACTS ABOUT OVARIAN CANCER

- Overall, the risk of ever getting ovarian cancer is small, about 1.4 percent for a woman without a family history.
- Ovarian cancer most commonly strikes women between the ages of 55 and 75.
- Over 90 percent of women with this cancer have *no* family history of it. And among those with a family history, nine out of ten have had only one affected relative.
- Women who have one first-degree relative (mother, sister, daughter) with this disease have a lifetime risk

of about 5 percent. With two relatives affected, the risk rises to 7 percent.

- The risk jumps to 50 percent or more for the 1 percent of women whose family histories include clusters of ovarian cancer over several generations (hereditary ovarian cancer syndrome), especially if their relatives had it at relatively young ages. Women in this group tend to be seven to fifteen years younger than the general population at the time of diagnosis. This high-risk group is currently under intense investigation in an effort to find genetic markers on chromosomes that can distinguish it from the nonhereditary variety. A genetic test for women in families known to be at special risk is expected momentarily.

- The risk rises when there are clusters of breast, uterine, prostate, or colon cancer in the family, because the same mutant gene may be causing a predisposition for all of these malignancies.

- Women who have been sterilized by having their tubes tied in a tubal ligation—the fallopian tubes are severed and cauterized—are only one-third as likely as other women to develop ovarian cancer, according to research by epidemiologists at Boston's Brigham and Women's Hospital. For that reason, some experts recommend the procedure for those who no longer want to have children and have a family history of ovarian cancer. Besides, sterilization is an excellent form of permanent contraception. No one knows why tubal ligation may reduce the risk of cancer, but the reason may be that the procedure diminishes the blood supply to the ovaries or that it causes a cancer-inhibiting hormonal change.

- A similar but smaller risk reduction is seen among women who have had hysterectomies but still have their ovaries.

"Why can't ovarian cancer be diagnosed early like other malignancies?"

Ovaries, normally about an inch in diameter, float in the abdominal cavity and can grow quite large before they may be detected in a pelvic examination. Even ultrasound can't always distinguish a cancer from a benign enlargement, and no test has yet been developed for the presence of ovarian cancer cells.

"What causes ovarian cancer?"

No specific causes have been found. We do know that there is a higher risk among women who have never been pregnant, especially if they have had unprotected sex for many years. And there is some evidence that a high-fat diet may raise the risk somewhat. In fact, women on complete vegetarian diets have been shown to have 40 percent less risk.

"Do fertility drugs cause it?"

It's most unlikely that they do, although infertile women (in fact, all women who have never been pregnant) have slightly increased risks of developing it. Even in the few studies that made fertility drugs look suspicious, there was no increased incidence of ovarian cancer among women who used fertility drugs and then became pregnant, but only among those who used them and did *not* get pregnant. So the truth may be that these women already had genetic abnormalities that prevented pregnancy and promoted cancer; see Chapter 10.

"This cancer scares me. Is there any way I could do something to prevent it?"

Consider taking birth-control pills. Many studies indicate that oral contraceptives may decrease the risk of ovarian cancer by about 50 percent. The protective effect increases with the length of time the pills are used and persists for ten to fifteen years after they have been abandoned.

Having babies helps, too. So does breastfeeding. Both pregnancy and breastfeeding, like oral contraceptives, result in less risk of ovarian cancer.

Eat a diet low in animal fats and high in fibrous vegetables, just in case it makes a difference. In any case, it's good for you.

And avoid using talcum powder on your genital area because there is some suspicion it may be an irritant that can raise the risk of ovarian cancer. You might try a powder made from cornstarch instead of talcum, but keep in mind that cornstarch may encourage fungal skin infections, especially in people with diabetes.

"How is ovarian cancer usually found?"

By accident. Early cases are most often discovered by chance during pelvic surgery that's performed for other reasons. Later cases do produce symptoms such as vague digestive disturbances, bloating, fatigue, and an increase in waist size.

"Can't the Pap smear detect it?"

The Pap test can detect cervical cancer, but provides no clues to ovarian cancer.

"What about other tests?"

Two screening methods are the best tests available so far, although they still aren't good enough. A National Institutes of Health medical panel recommends them only for women with hereditary syndromes that put them at high risk of ovarian cancer. Ever since the comedienne Gilda Radner died of this cancer in 1989, women have been urged to be tested, and many more women, fearful of cancer, have been demanding the procedures from their doctors. But, says the NIH panel, women who are not at high risk do not need routine screening and, in fact, take a chance of having unneeded surgery if they insist on having the tests whose results are unreliable.

The test that has generated the most publicity, the CA-125 blood test, which detects elevated levels of antibodies that have formed in response to cancer cells that are already present and have been shed by ovarian tumors, has been shown to miss at least half of all early tumors. What's more, it often registers positive because of conditions like pregnancy, menstruation, fibroids, liver disease, endometriosis, pelvic inflammatory disease, and other infections. By producing so many false positives, the CA-125 test is responsible for much unnecessary terror as well as surgery. It is, however, useful in women who have had ovarian cancer to see if a new cancer has developed.

Transvaginal ultrasound, the second technique, is being used more and more today to screen women with family histories of ovarian cancer for the presence of abnormal masses, although it too isn't always accurate. However, in its newest form—transvaginal color-flow Doppler ultrasonography—it has been found to pick up early tumors by detecting blood-vessel growth and measuring blood flow through the ovaries. New blood supply is associated with both benign and malignant masses, but the greatest vascular growth is almost always associated with malignancy. In addition, the greater the blood flow, the more likely the existence of cancer. This technique has been shown to be 96 percent accurate in distinguishing between malignant and nonmalignant masses and saves many women from emergency operations to remove their ovaries.

"I have a really frightening family history of ovarian cancer. Wouldn't it be best to have my ovaries removed before they cause trouble? I have three children and don't plan on any more."

That decision is easy if a skilled genetics counselor has determined that you have hereditary ovarian cancer syndrome, which gives you a 50 percent chance of getting ovarian cancer yourself. Then an oophorectomy is definitely warranted after you have completed your family.

If you don't have the syndrome but do have a cancer-prone family, then the answer is not so obvious. Having your ovaries removed means instant menopause and all of its consequences, from hot flashes to osteoporosis, so you must be prepared to take hormone replacement therapy to prevent premature aging and other problems.

"How are ovaries removed? Does it require a major operation?"

An oophorectomy is usually done by laparoscopy these days. This is a relatively simple "come and go" surgical procedure that requires only a small incision in the belly button and a couple of days of recovery time, although, of course, any operation has its risks.

Sometimes, however, the safest choice of surgical technique, especially if your uterus is to be removed at the same time, is an abdominal operation that involves a longer recovery but provides a better opportunity to check out the entire contents of your pelvic cavity. Remember, there's no sense in being "fashionable" when it comes to your well-being.

"I've read about taxol, a new anticancer drug. Isn't it a preventive or a treatment for ovarian cancer?"

Taxol was hailed as a miracle drug because it can dramatically shrink advanced ovarian cancers that recur after other chemotherapy. But the positive responses have proved to be temporary—some of the tumors grow again a few months after the treatment began. Taxol is nevertheless an important anticancer agent because, although it does not cure cancer, it slows its progress. Today it is being tested in combination with other drugs and with radiation therapy as well.

Earlier, taxol was in short supply because it was derived from the bark of the slow-growing Pacific yew tree, but it can now be synthesized in the laboratory.

Chapter 15

URINARY-TRACT INFECTIONS: HOW TO DEAL WITH THEM

IF YOU HAVE NEVER HAD A URINARY-TRACT INFECTION (UTI)—a most unpleasant ailment that gives you a painful burning sensation during urination and a bladder that continually demands to be emptied—you are an unusual and lucky woman. UTIs can afflict men, but they are primarily a woman's problem and many women suffer one bout after another. It has been estimated that at least half of all women have had at least one UTI (commonly called cystitis), and that 80 percent of this group has had them recurrently.

They are primarily a woman's disease because the female urethra, the tube that transports urine from the bladder, is very short—about 1.5 inches long, compared with 8 or 9 inches in men. In addition, its opening is located just above the vagina, where it is often traumatized during sexual intercourse, and it is close to the anus, where it can easily be contaminated with fecal material.

If that isn't enough, urethral tissue becomes less and less resistant to infection as the years go by and grows especially susceptible after menopause. The cause, once more, is the diminishing production of estrogen, the female hormone that is responsible for keeping vaginal and urethral tissue in good functioning condition.

Starting at around the age of 40, these tissues become less flexible and elastic with every passing year. After menopause, the urethral lining becomes thinner and more fragile, making it attractive territory for bacteria, while the distance between the vagina and the urethra becomes shorter, allowing infections to cross over from one to the other.

At the same time, because of a combination of aging and diminished estrogen, the bladder capacity is reduced as this inflatable organ becomes less elastic and its supports begin to sag. That's the major reason why you may not last through the night anymore without a trip or two to the bathroom. In addition, you—like many other women—probably sleep less soundly now and so are awakened more readily by a full bladder.

Another factor that can predispose to cystitis is a prolapsed vaginal wall that puts pressure on the urethra or the bladder and causes a tendency to allow residual urine to collect in the bladder, where an infection may then flourish.

If you are over 40 and have never had many UTIs in your earlier days but now seem to be getting them all the time, you can almost surely blame them on your altered anatomy and new hormonal status. But it is always possible that the UTIs recur for other reasons—perhaps a genetic predisposition, an obstruction such as a large fibroid, an abnormality in the urinary tract that doesn't allow the proper flow of urine, an immune problem, traumatic sexual practices, or poor personal hygiene. Don't try to figure this out on your own. See your doctor.

URINARY-TRACT INFECTIONS EXPLAINED

A UTI is an inflammation of the urinary tract usually caused by an invasion of bacteria and other organisms that normally live in the intestinal tract. It is called *urethritis* when it affects only the urethra, the narrow muscular tube that leads from the bladder to the outside of your body, and *cystitis* when the infection has reached the bladder. But for all practical purposes, it is known as cystitis if only because it is almost impossible to know just what part of the tract is inflamed, nor does it usually matter because the treatment is the same. However, if the infection involves the kidneys, then it is much more serious and changes its name to *pyelonephritis*.

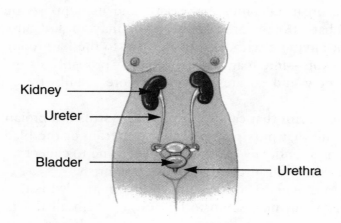

Kidney

Ureter

Bladder

Urethra

The invading bacteria enter through the urethra and then may travel upstream to the bladder or, unchecked, to the kidneys. Your first indication may be a feeling of irritation. Then, as the infection progresses, you will go on to a frequent and urgent need to urinate, a painful burning sensation during urination, sometimes accompanied by pain in the lower abdomen, back, or side, and cloudy, bloody, or even foul-smelling urine. In some cases these symptoms are accompanied by fever, chills, and nausea.

But sometimes the cystitis is silent. In other words, it is without symptoms and can be diagnosed only after a routine urine culture. And sometimes it is confused with vaginitis, an irritation of the vaginal area that may also cause a burning sensation when you urinate.

To get a proper diagnosis and treatment, you must see a doctor who will take a urine sample to screen for bacteria and will prescribe the appropriate antibiotic.

The Classic Symptoms of Cystitis

- Burning or pain when urinating
- Urgent need to urinate frequently, even when the output is small
- Painful sex
- Cloudy or bloody urine, sometimes foul-smelling

ARE UTIs PREVENTABLE?

Partially. There are a number of sensible, everyday ways to help fend off UTIs, but if you are constantly battling them you must take more aggressive measures, usually in the form of antibiotics. Here's what you can do:

- *Practice careful toilet habits.* In other words, remember what your mother taught you about wiping yourself from front to back, especially after a bowel movement. And wash this area of your body carefully and frequently (but don't be obsessive—too much soap and water can be drying). This can reduce the chance of infection by keeping bacteria away from both the urethra and the vagina.
- *Drink plenty of fluids.* Water is an excellent choice because it is cheap, available, and noncaloric, but anything liquid is fine for this purpose. Six or eight glasses a day should do it. Fluids flush out the urinary tract and dilute the

urine, making it less attractive to bacteria. Women who void infrequently are more likely to get a UTI because the urine is allowed to pool in the bladder, giving unfriendly organisms time to proliferate.

- *Drink cranberry or blueberry juice.* Although cranberry juice has been widely used as a folk remedy over the years, its effectiveness has only recently begun to be backed up by scientific evidence. A study at the Weizmann Institute of Science in Israel confirmed that, unlike other juices, both cranberry and blueberry juices can help prevent UTI because they contain compounds known to prevent bacteria from sticking to the walls of the bladder. How much should you drink? Nobody knows, but anywhere from 4 to 8 fluid ounces a day should be plenty. If your weight is a concern, drink low-calorie cranberry juice because the regular variety is loaded with sugar. As for blueberry juice, you may have to squeeze your own.

- *Eat more vegetables and fruits and fewer high-fat foods.* High-fat foods tend to produce a more alkaline urine, while a high-vegetable diet makes the urine more acid, the way it should be. A more acidic environment discourages the growth of bacteria.

- *Limit your alcohol consumption.* Alcohol dehydrates your body and concentrates the urine.

- *Try eliminating spicy foods and caffeine.* These sometimes act as irritants to the urethra, setting the stage for infections.

- *Wear underpants that are not too tight or binding.* Avoid panty hose and very tight jeans. Don't wear underpants to bed, either. Bacteria thrive in warm, moist, airless environments.

- *Change tampons or sanitary napkins frequently.* This will discourage the growth of bacteria.

- *Avoid vaginal douches or deodorants and perfumed soaps.* They tend to be irritating and drying, thereby issuing an invitation to urinary-tract infections. Besides, there is no legitimate reason for using them. If you feel compelled to douche, do it no more than once a week with plain warm water. Or to make the area more acid, use a mild solution of vinegar and water (1 tablespoon of white vinegar to 1 quart of warm water).

- *Don't hold it in.* Make a habit of urinating whenever you think of it, but always before you feel an urgent need to do so. Those who chronically hold it in increase their susceptibility to infection. Urinate before sexual intercourse, after sexual intercourse, before exercising, or before starting out on an automobile trip or a long shopping venture. Urinate as often as possible.
- *Make sure to empty your bladder.* Every time you use the toilet, empty your bladder completely. First thing in the morning, wait ten minutes after urinating and then urinate again.
- *Consider hormone replacement therapy.* Seriously think of beginning HRT if, after menopause, your problems with UTIs intensify. Even if you don't take estrogen systemically by pill or patch, you can use vaginal estrogen cream if only occasionally to thicken up both the vaginal and urethral tissues and make them less susceptible to infection.
- *Use a vaginal moisturizer.* Second choice (less effective than HRT) is one of the vaginal moisturizing creams, such as Replens or Gyne-Moistrin, that contain no hormones. One of their major attributes is that they are acidic (2.5 pH) and discouraging to bacteria.
- *Get used to new habits concerning sex* (see below).

"I am 58 and had menopause nine years ago. My doctor has suggested taking estrogen because of constant attacks of cystitis. Is this enough reason to start taking hormones?"

Yes, unless there is a valid reason in your case why you can't take them. Your UTIs are undoubtedly encouraged by urethral tissue that has become atrophic. Hormone replacement therapy can definitely help by restoring this tissue (as well as that of the vagina) to its former functional condition. It will also help return the pH of the vagina to a normal acidic state, reducing pathogenic vaginal flora and, as a result, the number of UTIs resulting from this source. In fact, HRT is frequently the only treatment that really works well for postmenopausal women; see Chapter 3.

"It seems like every time I have sexual intercourse, I get cystitis. It is very annoying, painful, and upsetting. Short of giving up sex, what can I do?"

Because sexual intercourse is notorious for causing UTIs by introducing bacteria at the opening of the urethra, try to follow a few simple rules:

1. Remember that physical trauma to the urethra during strenuous sexual activity is one of the most common causes of irritation and cystitis. All we can say here is try to go easy on these delicate parts of your anatomy.
2. Intercourse introduces bacteria from your skin and your partner's into the area. So be careful about your hygiene and his, and try to avoid sexual activities that may move bacteria from the anal area to the vagina. You are more likely, by the way, to get UTIs after intercourse with new partners, since it means possible exposure to new strains of infectious organisms. After a while, you become accustomed to the bacteria of a regular partner, a good argument for monogamy.
3. Be sure to empty your bladder before intercourse so it is less likely to suffer trauma. And more important, empty it immediately afterwards to wash out any bacteria that may have accumulated in the urethral area.
4. If you use a diaphragm, consider changing your method of contraception or have it checked for fit. A diaphragm that is the wrong size or positioned incorrectly can press against the neck of the bladder during intercourse, resulting in a backup of urine that serves as a breeding ground for bacteria. Because diaphragms must be left

in place for many hours after intercourse, the bacteria introduced into the bladder during sex may thus be given the opportunity to flourish. If you decide to continue using a diaphragm, don't leave it in any longer than necessary.

5. Spermicides have been accused of fostering UTIs because they can destroy the normal vaginal bacteria called lactobacilli but do not affect *E. coli,* the major cause of UTIs. Without the normal friendly bacteria, *E. coli* may colonize in the vagina and, during sex, move over to the urinary tract.

6. Use a water-soluble vaginal lubricant during intercourse. Do not use moisturizer or petroleum jelly or *anything* else except a lubricant made for this purpose because, instead of helping, it will only make matters worse (see Chapter 7).

7. If you always get a UTI after sex, ask your physician to prescribe a preventive antibiotic to be taken immediately before or after intercourse. A study of college women with a history of UTIs who took antibiotics within two hours of intercourse had only a 13 percent infection rate after six months, compared to an 82 percent rate among those who took placebos.

"What about taking lots of vitamin C to keep the urine acid? Isn't that supposed to help?"

It may help because acidic urine is not hospitable to bacteria. The problem is that you will have to take very large amounts to make a difference. Cranberry juice, too, is excreted as acid, another reason why it may help prevent infections. Citrus fruits, however, although they are acid when they enter the body, do not come out that way.

"I read that there's now a vaccine that will prevent urinary-tract infections. Since I get one infection after another, I'd be interested in trying it."

A Swiss-made vaccine is available in Europe but is still undergoing preliminary study in the United States. If it works, the vaccine—taken by vaginal suppository—should prevent many cases of UTI without the use of antibiotics, whose side effects may include yeast infections and allergic reactions. Bacteria can also become resistant to the drugs. The UTI vaccine stimulates production of antibodies that prevent bacteria from attaching to the bladder lining and initiating an infection.

WHAT YOU CAN DO *NOW*

Call your doctor immediately when you first notice that familiar burning sensation and the urge to empty your bladder every few minutes whether it's full or not. If your urine has not already been cultured for organisms, it should be now. The results of the culture test will not only identify the offending organism but also the antibiotic to which it is sensitive, and the doctor will start you on a course of treatment, usually a combination of sulfamethoxazole and trimethoprim such as Septra, or Bactrim, or Macrodantin. Noroxin is another antibiotic that may be prescribed as a second line of defense when the others fail to clear up the problem.

The regimens for antibiotic treatment vary and you and your doctor can decide which is best for you. Be sure to mention any allergies to antibiotics and keep in mind that the same kind of antibiotic can have several different brand names. Typical regimens are:

- *Bedtime preventive.* If you have frequent recurrent UTIs, you may do best with a small dose of an antibiotic either every night or every other night before you go to bed. Treat any resulting yeast infections with an antifungal medication.
- *Preventive before or after sex.* As we discussed earlier, a small dose of antibiotic taken just before or just after

intercourse may prevent UTIs that in your case inevitably follow sexual activity.

• *Single-dose or short-course treatment.* Most UTIs can be treated with either a single large dose of antibiotic or a relatively short course (three to ten days) of a standard dose. Infections involving the kidneys, however, may require much longer treatment. The disadvantage of the single dose is that the symptoms may persist for a couple of days after the treatment, while that of the longer course of treatment is that it may lead to vaginal yeast infections.

By the way, if you tend to get a yeast infection every time you take an antibiotic, buy one of the nonprescription antifungal medications such as Monistat or Gyne-Lotrimin and use it as a preventive for as long as you take the antibiotic.

Concurrent with your antibiotic therapy, these home remedies may help speed recovery when you get a UTI:

1. Be sure to take *all* of the prescribed medication even if you feel better and your symptoms have gone away. A partial dose does not necessarily kill all the bacteria and may create resistant strains, so finishing the prescription is essential if you are not looking for a recurrence.

2. Drink plenty of fluids to dilute the bacteria and flush out the bladder.

3. Drink 8 ounces of cranberry or blueberry juice a day.

4. Avoid alcohol, coffee, tea, or caffeinated soft drinks.

5. Urinate frequently, without waiting for the urge.

6. To help relieve discomfort, apply heat to the bladder area with a heat lamp or a heating pad set low.

7. Ask your physician to give you a prescription for antibiotics in advance and keep it on hand, especially when you travel, so you can begin treatment the moment you start feeling the symptoms. It's amazing how many UTIs seem to start on weekends.

IC: THE OTHER KIND OF CYSTITIS

A very different and much more troublesome kind of cystitis plagues over a half-million Americans, 90 percent of them women. Called *interstitial cystitis* (IC), it is not a bacterial infection but an inflammatory disease of the bladder wall with symptoms that start out similar to those of common UTIs but become much worse. Unlike UTIs, IC does not respond to antibiotics. Dismissed for years as a psychosomatic female ailment, IC has only recently been recognized as a real disease with devastating effects.

Characterized by severe pain and the incessant urge to urinate, interstitial cystitis has no known cause or cure. In severe cases, a woman with IC suffers intractable pain and must make a trip to the bathroom every twenty minutes, day and night, often leading to chronic sleep deprivation and depression.

In general, the symptoms of IC vary from mild to severe, from intermittent to constant, often with acute flareups and temporary remissions. Among the 10 percent of people with classic IC, the most serious type, the bladder lining is covered with tiny pinpoint hemorrhages, ulcers, and scarring, and the bladder itself contracts so it holds less and less fluid. In the more common nonulcer type, the hemorrhages, or glomerulations, are present but the bladder capacity may remain near normal.

For helpful information, contact:

The Interstitial Cystitis Foundation
P.O. Box 1553
Madison Square Station
New York, New York 10159
212-979-6057

"What causes interstitial cystitis?"

There are lots of theories but no real answers. The possibilities include a defect in the normally protective bladder lining, an abnormality in the bladder structure, an autoimmune reaction, toxic or irritating substances in the urine, and neurogenic inflammation.

"How is it diagnosed?"

When a complete urinary workup comes out negative, ruling out bacterial infections, sexually transmitted diseases, endometriosis, cancer, and other possibilities, the next step is close examination of the bladder lining by cystoscopy. The bladder is inspected with a fiberoptic probe that may reveal inflammation and pinpoint hemorrhages on the bladder wall, the hallmarks of this disease. A biopsy may then be made to rule out bladder cancer and help diagnose IC.

"Are there treatments for IC?"

About a third of IC patients report relief from the cystoscopy itself. In addition, there are many treatments available, although none of them works for everyone. They include DMSO (dimethyl sulfoxide), bladder distention, antidepressants such as amitriptyline (Elavil), transcutaneous electrical nerve stimulation (TENS), and other drugs, many of them still experimental. Surgery (cystoplasty) is a last resort.

Chapter 16

INCONTINENCE: THE BIG SECRET

ADMITTING TO URINARY INCONTINENCE is more difficult for many women than revealing their incomes or discussing their problems in bed. It's humiliating to let anyone know your most intimate secret: that you occasionally lose control of your bladder and wet your pants. Although you may think you're the only adult around with this embarrassing problem, you have plenty of company, most of whom are equally reluctant to talk about it.

Millions of Americans of all ages and both sexes suffer from incontinence, all the way from an occasional minor leak during sex or a sneeze to such a major lack of control that they hesitate to leave home for fear of having an accident.

Up to 26 percent of adult women are incontinent to some degree, experts estimate, and as many as 40 percent of women over 45 have the problem at least occasionally. Women are three to five times more likely to have leaky bladders than men, particularly if they have had children, and the incidence rises rapidly with age. Up to 66 percent of people over 60 have been afflicted with incontinence at one time or another;

in fact, uncontrollable bladders are a primary reason why old people end up in nursing homes.

The shame of it is that almost everyone with this problem could be significantly improved or even cured with the proper treatment. It's not normal to be incontinent, no matter how old you are. Not a disease but a symptom of an underlying condition that can usually be corrected or mitigated, incontinence can be caused by such things as recurrent infections, lack of estrogen after menopause, weak pelvic muscles, a sagging bladder, large fibroids, muscle damage during childbirth, obesity, pelvic surgery, even severe constipation. Treat those conditions and your problem may well be solved.

The Urinary Tract

The urinary tract consists of the kidneys; ureters, two long tubes to the bladder; the bladder, which stores the urine produced in the kidneys; and the urethra, the passageway from the bladder to the outside of the body, that emerges very close to the opening of the vagina.

WHAT YOU CAN DO *NOW*

Most women with leaky bladders have never been treated for their problem. They don't mention it to their doctors and often their doctors don't ask them if they have it. One survey, in fact, found that people wait an average of nine years before seeking help. Left untreated, urinary incontinence can make life miserable. So the first thing to do is to tell your doctor about it and to have a thorough examination. Your primary physician or gynecologist may feel competent to treat you or may send you on to a specialist—a urologist or a urogynecologist.

The second step is to devote yourself to working at solving your problem. Many treatments are available, ranging from simple things you can do at home to drugs and surgery. The usual introductory measure is a program of pelvic exercises that are easy and simple but require self-discipline and take a bit of time to show real results.

The treatment that is appropriate for you depends on the kind and degree of incontinence you have as well as the reason you have it. Almost all cases of incontinence among older women are caused by the first two (or a combination of the two) of the following basic types:

- *Stress incontinence.* The most common variety, it allows an involuntary spurt of urine when all you're doing is sneezing, coughing, laughing, lifting, exercising, or standing up quickly. It can also happen when you're having sexual intercourse. Usually caused by a weakened urethral sphincter or a sagging urethra that allows urine to seep out when the abdomen exerts pressure on the bladder, it tends to get worse after menopause when your estrogen level drops off. This sagging or prolapse of the urethra is often accompanied by prolapse of the bladder, rectum, or uterus, and happens most frequently in women who delivered their children vaginally.
- *Urge incontinence.* Harder to deal with is a bladder that contracts without your permission at inopportune moments. It is the uncontrollable urge to go to the toilet with too little warning and the failure to get there on time. This usually results from infection, inflammation, or damage that leads to oversensitivity of the nerves and muscles, causing the bladder to become spastic or unstable.
- *Overflow incontinence.* In this less common type, the bladder outlet (sphincter) becomes resistant to flow and the bladder doesn't empty completely. When more urine is produced than the bladder can hold, it overflows in little dribbles.

• *Reflex incontinence.* With this variety, you are unaware that your bladder is full because of nerve damage, frequently from diabetes, that impairs the ability to sense the need to void.

WHY YOU LOSE CONTROL

Among the many causes of a bladder (the elastic, muscular holding tank capable of storing eight to sixteen ounces of urine) that doesn't behave the way you'd like it to are:

• **Age and menopause:** Like many other parts of the body, the lower urinary tract—the bladder and urethra (the tube that carries urine from the bladder out of the body)— changes as you get older. The muscle of the bladder outlet tends to lose some of its tone and the bladder wall becomes stiffer, diminishing its ability to expand.

Add to that the effects of menopause. With the loss of female hormones, the bladder loses even more muscle tone and elasticity, making it less able to hold as much urine as it once did. The outermost portion of the urethra also becomes less flexible and elastic, and therefore becomes more subject to injury and infection. The urethral lining thins and weakens so it may no longer keep the bladder closed when you're not urinating. Not only that, but the shrinking walls of the vagina after menopause provide less support for the fragile urethra. Sometimes in severe cases of estrogen deficiency, the urethra prolapses, sagging into the vagina, so that a sneeze or a jolt is all you need to precipitate an "accident."

Obviously, not all postmenopausal women become incontinent, although you will certainly notice you're making more trips to the bathroom than you ever did before. But lack of female hormones can be enough to tip the balance if you are already susceptible to the problem for other reasons.

- **Weakened pelvic muscles:** The pelvic floor—the muscles that encircle and support the urethra, vagina, and rectum—often become stretched and less supportive because of pregnancies, childbirth, previous surgery, normal aging, and a lack of estrogen. When, as a result, the bladder and urethra drop lower in the pelvis where they press against other organs, they become less able to hold urine under pressure. A prolapsed bladder is called a cystocele, and a sagging urethra a urethracele.
- **Urinary tract infections:** When the bladder is infected, it may become extremely irritated, which causes it to contract, making it less able to hold back urine.
- **Obesity:** Being vastly overweight increases abdominal pressure on the bladder.
- **Medications and foods:** Medications such as antihypertensives and antidepressants, and foods such as sugar, coffee, alcohol, artificial sweeteners, and spicy dishes, sometimes cause incontinence as a side effect, especially when muscles and sphincters are weakened for other reasons.
- **Pelvic surgery:** Muscles and nerves, and even the organs themselves, may be damaged during earlier surgery. Although this is rare, it can be the cause of incontinence when the sensory nerves of the bladder are cut or the bladder is bruised or torn.

"I never had any problems with my bladder before menopause. Why can't I exercise anymore without having an accident? I'm always running for the bathroom and very often I don't make it."

The estrogen-depleted bladder lacks elasticity, holds less urine, is easily traumatized, and becomes less resistant to infection and inflammation. The mucosa around the urethra shrinks, resulting in a nonwatertight seal at its outlet. Blood flow to the area decreases. The muscles within and around the bladder and the urethra, as well as the supports holding it in place, become more relaxed, exacerbating the effect of having had vaginal deliveries that permanently stretch the pelvic tissues. All of these factors combine to lower the ability of the bladder and urethra to hold back urine when you run around, jump, or even have a good laugh.

"So won't hormone replacement therapy help the problem?"

It will definitely help, but it may not cure you. Estrogen replacement is the first line of treatment to consider when you have stress and/or urge incontinence because it can restore the bladder and urethral tissue to a state that's a lot closer to its former self.

"I hesitate to take estrogen because it's supposed to be dangerous. Will taking progesterone alone help?"

No, estrogen is what you need. HRT is not dangerous if there's no medical reason why you can't take it and if you take it in a correct and cautious way (see Chapter 3). If you don't want to take estrogen systemically, ask your doctor to prescribe vaginal estrogen cream. Applied topically, the cream's effects are almost completely limited to the vagina and the urethra, relieving the atrophy and with it, in simple cases, the leaking.

"How come I lose control of my bladder when I have intercourse? This is extremely embarrassing."

Although this is something women rarely admit even to their doctors, it happens to an amazing number of women. Most leak urine with penetration and some with orgasm. The reason is that intercourse and orgasm are simply other ways of applying pressure to a bladder that's none too flexible anymore and to a urethral sphincter that no longer closes tightly because of thinning tissues. Estrogen treatment may be helpful unless the urethra and bladder have already sagged too far, in which case surgery may be needed.

What's an irritable bladder? That's what my doctor says I have."

It's when only a small amount of urine makes the bladder feel full and you feel an urgent need to void. Often avoiding certain foods and other substances that make it irritable, such as alcohol, caffeine, chocolate, and some medications, can help.

"How does diabetes affect the bladder?"

The peripheral nerves associated with the bladder muscles are sometimes damaged by diabetes or other diseases that affect the nerves, so the bladder may not recognize when it is full. It becomes overextended and releases urine under stress.

"I have always been constipated and have been told that this could be the reason for my bladder problem. Why would this be so?"

When you strain to have a bowel movement, you increase the intra-abdominal pressure dramatically, putting pressure on what may already be weakened bladder and urethral tissues.

"Are there any tricks to holding back urine when you sneeze or cough?"

To avoid wet pants and a red face, try contracting the pelvic floor muscles very hard whenever you feel a sneeze or cough coming on. Or, sitting down, cross one leg completely over the other and bend at the waist.

"I try to drink as little fluid as possible so I won't have an accident, but that doesn't seem to help. Why not?"

If you let yourself become chronically dehydrated, the urine you do produce will be so concentrated and irritating to the bladder that it can cause a constant urge to get to the bathroom fast. Exactly what you don't need.

WHAT TO DO ABOUT INCONTINENCE

The doctor will make a diagnosis of your problem and its cause by giving you a complete physical and neurological examination, a urinalysis to check for infection, bladder-function tests, and perhaps a cystoscopy. Cystoscopy is a close examination of the bladder and urethra with the help of a lighted instrument that is passed through the urethra. You may be asked to keep a diary for a few days, noting your trips to the bathroom, the amount of urine voided, episodes of incontinence, the food you eat, the activities you engage in, and the medications you take.

Although your primary physician may have the expertise to perform some or all of these tests, in most cases you will be referred to a specialist, usually a urologist. Be sure to see a specialist who has extensive expertise in incontinence; many gynecologists are too quick to offer surgery as the only solution.

Then a treatment program will be prescribed, depending, of course, on the cause of the problem. Sometimes simple changes in diet or the elimination of certain drugs can cure you or at least greatly improve the situation. Often clearing up an infection with antibiotics will do it. Sometimes the problem is solved by behavioral techniques such as bladder training, muscle-strengthening exercises, biofeedback, or frequent trips to the toilet. Other treatments include medications to increase bladder capacity, relax the bladder, or stimulate contractions. Only in extreme or intransigent cases is surgery warranted.

Almost always, a combination of treatments and self-help measures is used. Keep the faith because, although it can take a few months, the results can be impressive and you may see a remarkable improvement if you work at it. Here are the usual treatments:

- *Estrogen replacement.* HRT is usually used in combination with other kinds of therapy although, by itself, it may do the trick if your problem is mild. And it is frequently prescribed for about six months before pelvic surgery to restore the tissues to their optimal condition before the operation.
- *Bladder training.* Bladder training teaches you to urinate at scheduled times only, with gradually increasing intervals between trips to the toilet.

  It usually works this way: You start off by going to the toilet by the clock every thirty to sixty minutes during the day, whether or not you feel the need, resisting urges at unscheduled times by relaxing or distracting yourself, and then voiding on schedule. After a few days or a week, you increase the time between trips by half an hour, continuing to increase it by half-hour increments every week or so until, after about six weeks, you have trained your bladder to wait at least four hours.
- *Kegel exercises.* Designed to strengthen the muscles supporting the base of the bladder and give you control over your body, these exercises can often do wonders for incontinence, especially the stress variety. You must first get the feel of tightening the proper muscles, the same ones that are used to stop the flow of urine in midstream.

  Whenever you think of it, as many times a day as possible (start off slowly and gradually increase the episodes), tighten the muscles as if you were trying very hard to hold back your urine. Keep your abdomen, buttocks, and thigh muscles relaxed. Tighten, hold for ten seconds, relax, at least twenty times per session.

The virtue of these exercises is that nobody can tell you're doing them so you can do them whenever you like, at a party, in the car, at the movies, during a business meeting. But don't expect quick results. It usually takes a few months of faithful exercising to strengthen the muscles enough to make your sphincter more watertight. And then you must keep it up. Stop exercising and the muscles relax again.

Here's another way to accomplish the same thing: Sit on the toilet with a full bladder, start to urinate, then tighten up to stop the flow. Holding back, count slowly to 10. Repeat up to twenty times. Now finish.

For women who have trouble finding their pelvic-floor muscles, there are special weighted vaginal cones designed for this purpose. The plastic cones, used in gradually increasing weights, are inserted into the vagina. Then, in your efforts to hold them in, you train yourself to tighten the appropriate muscles.

Biofeedback training, perhaps combined with electrical stimulation, can also help you learn how to contract the proper muscles and to urinate only at the appropriate signal.

• *Double-voiding*. Because it is important to empty your bladder completely when you urinate, which is difficult for many women, get in the habit of voiding, waiting a few minutes, then going again. Or stand up, bend over, walk around, perhaps rub your lower abdomen, then sit down and finish the job.

• *Medications*. Drugs can increase the bladder's ability to hold urine by decreasing its involuntary urges or by tightening the sphincter muscle. Some are designed to block involuntary bladder contractions. Another decreases urine production. Others are used to reduce bladder wall contractions or tighten the sphincter muscles around the urethra. And still others help relax the bladder sphincter.

Often, these medications work best when they are used in combination with hormone replacement therapy.

• *Treatment for infection.* Other medications such as antibiotics can eradicate underlying infections that may be the culprit.

• *Drug avoidance.* Some prescribed medications, including several used to control hypertension, have been linked with leakage problems. Check yours out with your doctor. Others that can cause trouble for susceptible women are sedatives, diuretics, antidepressants, antihistamines, and decongestants.

• *Periurethral injections.* Promising but not yet approved by the FDA, the injection of synthetic materials such as collagen around the urethra has been found to support and compress it by creating a mound of tissue that allows the urethra to close up again.

• *Surgery.* If all else fails, surgery can be remarkably effective. It can correct structural abnormalities, reposition a sagging bladder and urethra, strengthen the supports, remove obstructions, bolster weakened muscles, replace a defective sphincter, and remove large fibroids that obstruct the bladder or urethra.

HOW TO HELP YOURSELF

Meanwhile, there are a number of things *you* can do to help yourself avoid, improve, or cure a misbehaving bladder.

1. Consume a lot of liquids. You may be cutting back on your fluid intake hoping that you won't have to go to the toilet so often. But the smaller amount of urine you produce when you are dehydrated may be more highly concentrated, which makes it irritating to the bladder and more likely to encourage bacterial infections. Don't cut back unless instructed to do so by your doctor.

2. Learn to empty your bladder completely and keep it as empty as possible. As one droll gynecologist advises,

"Never pass a toilet without making a contribution," even if you don't have a strong urge to go.

3. Lose some pounds if you are considerably overweight. A loss of 5 to 10 percent of body weight sometimes helps enormously to take the pressure off your urinary tract.

4. Ditch the cigarettes. Women who smoke have more than double the risk of urinary incontinence than nonsmokers, says a recent study. Smoking not only irritates the bladder lining and perhaps damages the sphincter nerves but is associated with bladder cancer. It also makes you cough, which could lead to leaks.

4. Try eliminating the following foods that are bladder irritants for many people: alcohol, carbonated beverages, caffeine, milk, citrus, tomatoes, spicy foods, sugar, honey, chocolate, artificial sweeteners.

5. Avoid colored or perfumed toilet paper and feminine hygiene products, detergent bath additives, and perfumed soaps.

6. Eat a high-fiber diet to prevent constipation. Consuming lots of fruits and vegetables is also thought to help prevent bladder cancer.

7. Never strain during a bowel movement.

8. Don't make a habit of ignoring the urge to defecate.

9. Avoid heavy lifting, which puts a strain on the structural supports of the pelvic floor.

You can get useful information, a guide to products and services, a newsletter, and answers to questions from:

HIP (Help for Incontinent People, Inc.)
P.O. Box 544
Union, South Carolina 29379
800-BLADDER or 803-579-7900

"Do I have to keep on doing the Kegel exercises forever or can I quit after I stop having problems?"

Keep them up because it doesn't take long for muscles that are not exercised to become weak all over again.

"What do I do if the exercises and other everyday measures don't work?"

If there's no significant improvement after a couple of months of faithful squeezing and clean living, go back to your doctor and discuss other treatments. Or perhaps even better, ask for a referral to a specialist. You could see some improvement in two or three weeks or it could take up to six months to accomplish the optimum results.

"I have an even more embarrassing problem than leaking urine. Whenever I have loose bowels, I leak stool. What do I do about that?"

The same kind of exercises—tightly contracting the anal sphincter muscles as often as possible—can usually strengthen them enough to allow you to hold back more easily. Check with your doctor to see if there is nerve or muscle damage to the rectal sphincter.

Chapter 17

YOUR COLON: AVOIDING CANCER AND OTHER PROBLEMS

HAVING A RECTAL EXAMINATION and making stool smears are certainly not among anybody's favorite activities. But if you can save your life by overcoming your reluctance to undergo these indignities once a year, it's certainly worth the momentary discomfort. "Don't die of embarrassment" is how the American Cancer Society puts it.

Among internal malignancies, colon cancer is second only to lung cancer as a cause of death in the United States for both women and men. About 150,000 new cases are now diagnosed every year, with about 60,000 of them, almost all over the age of 50, dying as a result. The risk increases with age. That makes it something to be concerned about, especially when it may be preventable and can certainly be cured when it's caught early.

WHO GETS COLON CANCER?

You are in special danger of developing cancer of the colon or rectum if any of the following predisposing factors apply to you:

- *Family history*. If you have a first-degree relative (parent, sibling, or child) who has had colon cancer, you have a risk two to three times higher than the average woman of getting it.
- *Genetic susceptibility*. As many as 1 in every 200 people, or more than a million Americans, is thought to be a carrier of a defective gene that greatly increases the risk of colon cancer and a handful of other cancers as well. This familial disorder, called *hereditary nonpolyposis colon cancer*, accounts for up to 15 percent of all colon cancers. A blood test for it, expected to be available momentarily, will allow people who harbor the trait to take preventive action.
- *Familial adenomatous polyposis (FAP)*. Much less common is FAP, another genetic disorder, that affects 1 in 7,000 Americans. FAP patients develop hundreds, sometimes thousands of polyps, in the colon and rectum in their early teens and almost invariably develop cancer by age 40 if left untreated. This rare genetic susceptibility, passed along to half of the children of a parent with FAP, requires frequent exams and diligent removal of the polyps.

  Scientists at the Johns Hopkins University School of Medicine have developed a simple diagnostic blood test to pinpoint people who harbor this rare mutant gene that makes them almost certain to develop colon cancer. This means that a person who has inherited the gene can choose a course of heightened vigilance and anti-inflammatory drugs, while a family member shown to be free of it can stop worrying about it.

- *Ulcerative colitis.* A woman with a ten-year history of colitis—chronic inflammation of the large intestine—has a risk ratio of about twenty times that of the average woman for developing colon cancer.
- *Crohn's disease.* This is a chronic inflammatory disease of the gastrointestinal tract, usually the ileum, that may be an immune-deficiency disease. Your risk of colon cancer after ten years is only slightly lower than that for ulcerative colitis.

WHAT YOU CAN DO *NOW*

If you make a few simple lifestyle changes (*and* have regular checkups), you can make a significant difference in your chances of developing colon cancer:

1. *Eat more vegetables, fruits, and grains.* There's strong evidence that a high-fiber diet can significantly reduce the risk of colon cancer, especially if your fruits and vegetables contain folic acid.
2. *Drink plenty of liquids.* This helps your food to pass through more quickly.
3. *Cut down on dietary fat.* Although there is no definitive proof that high-fat diets can cause this cancer, more and more experts agree that the likelihood is that it can.
4. *Take low-dose aspirin regularly.* If you are at special risk, consider taking aspirin. Some experts claim that the chance of fatal colon cancer is cut up to half by those who use aspirin at least sixteen times a month for a year or more. Aspirin (unfortunately, nobody yet knows the optimal dose) is believed to inhibit polyp formation and runaway cell growth.
5. *Lose a few pounds if you are overweight.* Obesity has been linked to colon cancer.
6. *Get regular exercise.* Although the connection hasn't been

firmly established, many studies have examined the relationship between physical activity and colon cancer, and have concluded that sitting around on your duff increases the risk. One reason may be that exercise helps speed waste through the colon, giving it less time to make toxic contact with the lining.

7. *Take calcium supplements.* Not only are they good for your bones, but researchers have shown calcium supplements may be good for your colon, too.

8. *Take antioxidant vitamins.* Some studies suggest that vitamins A, C, E—vitamins that reduce the formation of free radicals—will also decrease the incidence of colon cancer. A joint Chinese and American study also included selenium. While all this remains to be proved conclusively, using vitamin supplements presents little risk and a potential gain.

9. *Consume more folic acid.* Folic acid, a vitamin in the B family, may be a significant factor in the prevention of colon cancer and may play a part in the process that switches off cancer genes. A Harvard Medical School study suggests that a high intake of folic acid from fresh fruits and vegetables and vitamin supplements is associated with lower risk.

10. *Watch for warning signs.* Don't ignore any of the following: rectal bleeding, blood in the stool, persistent narrowing of the stool, an urgent and painful need to defecate, or a persistent change in bowel habits. If you have any of these warning signs, pick up the telephone and make an appointment with your doctor to check them out. And even if you don't, you must have regular physical exams that include stool tests (see below).

"What are polyps? Why should we worry about them?"

Polyps are not cancer, but some of them are premalignant, which means that left alone they may eventually change into cancer. They are overgrowths of connective tissue and mucus membrane attached to the intestinal lining by short sometimes flexible stems that tend to announce themselves by minor bleeding. Most often, however, they issue no warning sign at all.

"Should a polyp always be removed?"

Yes, because it may be premalignant. A recent study by researchers at seven major medical centers reported that removal of polyps cuts the colon cancer rate by 90 percent. Polyps tend to recur, so if you've had them, a colonoscopy once a year is an excellent idea. If you've never had polyps but they run in your family, a colonoscopy every three years is considered sufficient.

"What causes rectal bleeding?"

The hidden blood found in a stool test or visible blood in the toilet bowl almost always comes from benign causes such as hemorrhoids. Nevertheless, any bleeding *must* be investigated and the cause identified because there is no sense taking a chance that it comes from polyps or early cancer.

"What's the safest way to deal with constipation, a problem that plagues everyone in our family?"

Don't take laxatives. Don't take enemas. Instead, eat a diet high in fiber, accompanied by at least eight glasses of fluid a day. That means lots of fruits and vegetables and grains. A bowl of high-fiber cereal topped with prunes every morning can do wonders. Other helpful habits: increase your physical activity; try to have a bowel movement soon after a meal, preferably breakfast; use a low step stool for your feet while sitting on the toilet.

SCHEDULE FOR A HEALTHY COLON

Cancer of the colon is completely curable when it's found early. Neglected, however, it can spread and become a killer. Here's what you and your doctor can do to reduce your chances of getting it in the first place:

- *All ages.* Your annual physical examination should include a thorough evaluation of your colon—a routine digital rectal exam and a test for blood in the stool. Virtually all colon cancers start out from benign but precancerous growths (polyps) on the lining of the bowel, which usually cause no noticeable symptoms at all. If the routine exam turns up anything suspicious, you will be sent for further tests.

  If you have a family history of colon cancer, put yourself in the hands of a specialist who will test you regularly for early signs of cancer.
- *Over 40.* If you are over 40, high risk or not, a sigmoidoscopy should also be included as part of your checkup for two consecutive years and, if it comes out negative, every two to three years thereafter. And if you are over 40 and/or have an increased risk of this kind of cancer, add a colonoscopy to the list every three to five years.

EARLY DETECTION: HOW IT'S DONE

Today there are several good screening techniques for detecting the presence of polyps or early symptomless cancers before they cause big trouble.

DIGITAL EXAM

The simplest screening test is a physical examination of the rectum. The doctor inserts a gloved finger into the rectum and feels for growths. Maybe uncomfortable, but seldom painful and always quick.

FECAL OCCULT BLOOD TEST

Because the physician can reach only a small portion of the colon, the rectal exam is always coupled with a test that detects the presence of hidden blood. Between them, the digital exam and the blood test pick up 40 to 50 percent of colon cancers.

Simple and inexpensive, the fecal occult blood test involves smearing tiny samples of your stool on a prepared test card after three consecutive bowel movements. The smears are then tested by the physician or a laboratory, using a chemical that reacts to traces of blood by turning blue. If blood is present in any of the samples, the test is considered positive.

About 1 percent of stool tests come out positive, but because the test is not specific for cancer, you may well get a false-positive result that requires further investigation. The fact is that only about one out of six people with positive results turns out to have an anatomic abnormality, benign or malignant.

Some Don'ts Before the Test

Positive results to the stool test are usually due to benign conditions—such as hemorrhoids or ulcers—that are a lot less frightening than cancer, so don't assume the worst when your doctor tells you further investigation is needed. False positives can also be traced to what you've taken into your digestive tract immediately before the testing.

So, for at least two days before the test and on the days you are making the stool samples, avoid the following:

- Vitamin C or foods rich in vitamin C because it may produce a false-negative result by preventing the chemical test from reacting to blood.
- Aspirin or other nonsteroidal anti-inflammatory drugs because they can make the stomach or intestine bleed. These should be avoided for a week before the test.
- Red meat because animal hemoglobin also tests positive.
- Foods that contain peroxidase, an enzyme that reacts positively to the testing chemical: broccoli, cauliflower, melons, radishes, turnips, horseradish.

FLEXIBLE SIGMOIDOSCOPY

Recommended for women over 40 as a routine addition to an annual checkup, a sigmoidoscopy gives the physician a good view of about a third of your entire colon. Tipped with a light and a lens, the two-foot-long fiberoptic flexible sigmoidoscope is inserted into the rectum and is carefully pushed along through the colon. The usual preparation is two Fleet enemas on the morning of the exam.

A sigmoidoscopy takes about five minutes, does not require a sedative, and usually doesn't cause real pain. On the other hand, it can be quite uncomfortable and is never on anyone's list of wonderful experiences.

COLONOSCOPY

The most effective test, colonoscopy allows a close look at the lining of your entire colon, all five feet of it. It uses a much longer flexible fiberoptic instrument with direct light transmission and is threaded through the rectum all the way through the twists and folds in the colon to the cecum. In the hands of a trained practitioner, in most cases a gastroenterologist, it allows better than 95 percent of malignant and benign growths to be identified.

The colonoscope provides another service as well. Because it is hollow, a surgical instrument can be inserted through it to take biopsies or remove polyps that are spotted along the way.

Too sophisticated and too expensive to be used routinely as a screening procedure, colonoscopy is prescribed only as a follow-up for the other tests and for screening high-risk candidates for colon cancer. The preparation the night before the examination usually involves a liquid diet for a day and drinking a special salt solution the night before to clean out the entire bowel. A colonoscopy is usually done under sedation in an office or hospital outpatient procedure.

BARIUM ENEMA

Another technique for examining the colon is the barium enema, not used for routine screening but as an alternative diagnostic procedure when the results of other tests come out positive. In some ways, it is more useful than colonoscopy because it reveals the contours of the outside of the colon walls as well as the lining, allowing extrinsic irregularities such as hernias and diverticulae to show up. On the other hand, it is purely diagnostic and any polyps or ulcers that are found will have to be removed during a subsequent colonoscopy.

As you must suspect, you are given an enema that fills your rectum and colon with barium, a radio-opaque fluid. Then a visualization of the lining is displayed on a fluoroscope, showing any distortions, growths, or ulcerations. The whole procedure takes anywhere from thirty minutes to an hour.

A barium enema requires a thoroughly cleansed bowel and may be very uncomfortable because the pressure of the incoming liquid—sometimes supplemented by gas—inflates and distends the colon. It, too, allows 90 to 95 percent of growths to be identified.

Chapter 18

LOOKING GOOD: YOUR SKIN, HAIR, NAILS

YOUR SKIN SERVES NOT ONLY TO WRAP YOU UP, hold you together, and protect your body from leakage and invasion, but along with your hair and nails, it is the part of you that shows. As your outermost layer and initial presentation to the world, it provides the most obvious reminder—to you and everybody else—of the passage of time.

Women feel considerable pressure—internal and external—to look good, whatever their age, and many spend enormous amounts of time and money trying to preserve, camouflage, or repair their outsides. There's certainly nothing wrong with that if reason and realism prevail because looking good can certainly help you feel positive about yourself.

But your skin's health is even more important, only partly because its condition is reflected in its appearance. The skin, the amazingly tough protective covering that envelops you, is the body's largest organ and one of its most complex. It marks the borders of your personal territory, acts as a buffer between you and the environment, and performs a broad range of essential biological functions. Every square inch of your skin contains several feet of blood vessels, hundreds of oil and sweat glands, over a thousand nerve endings, and millions of cells.

Although all skin undergoes normal aging over time and shows it eventually, many changes can be attributed to the cumulative effects of a lifetime of abuse and neglect, especially among the generation of women now in their middle years, who spent their youths in pursuit of a deep tan. Although you can't undo the past, you can lessen its impact, repair some of the damage, and avoid new assaults by treating your skin with respect, now and ever after.

HOW THE SKIN AGES

As the skin grows older, it doesn't fit as well, it doesn't look as good, and it isn't as comfortable. Gradually losing moisture, elasticity, fat, and mass, it becomes more fragile and less resistant to disease, slower to heal, more prone to bruising, and less able to regulate body temperature.

In the meantime, blood supply diminishes and the ability of its cells to renew themselves declines until, at age 60, they take twice as long to replace themselves as they did when you were young. Now the cells of the *epidermis*, the surface layer of the skin, no longer remain lined up in the nice, neat, orderly rows that produce young smooth skin. Instead it starts to become disorganized and irregularly arranged. Its cells tend to accumulate on the surface and are shed more slowly.

Moisture content, oil production, and sweat dwindle and the underlying support structure weakens. The subcutaneous fat layer shrinks while collagen fibers, the connective tissue in the *dermis* (the underlying layer), gradually decrease in number, organization, and density. Elastin—the elastic fibers woven into the collagen—becomes less resilient. Meanwhile, the number and function of the pigment cells decrease, fat tissue drops to the lower part of the face, sabaceous glands enlarge, and the muscles beneath the skin shrink.

That's the bad news. The good news is that, by carefully protecting your skin and taking meticulous care of it, you can hold off many of these aging changes for years longer than your careless peers.

WHY THE SKIN AGES

According to Wendy Keller Epstein, M.D., Assistant Clinical Professor of Dermatology at New York University School of Medicine, there are both intrinsic and extrinsic factors involved in all of these happenings: your genes, your hormones, and the amount of abuse to which you have subjected yourself.

THE INTRINSIC FACTORS

Normal chronological aging appears to be genetically programmed, so study your closest older relatives to get an idea of what you are likely to look like at their age if you live more or less under the same conditions. In general, very fair skin shows its age much more and much earlier than dark skin, which is protected by more pigment. The intrinsic aging changes, mainly a slowdown in cell renewal, do not become apparent in protected skin until your fifties or sixties. But when the changes are accelerated by environmental damage, they can make an unwelcome appearance decades earlier.

Female hormones play a significant role in determining how well your skin fares. Estrogen is largely responsible for the distribution of subcutaneous fat, the layer of fat just under the epidermis that provides inner support, firmness, and resilience. It helps to maintain moisture in the tissues by stimulating the production of hyaluronic acid, which holds water. And it encourages the formation of collagen, the connective tissue that keeps the skin thick and firm.

That's why you'll notice many skin changes in the first few years after menopause. In fact, a recent British study reported that the condition of the skin correlates more closely with how many years you have spent without estrogen than with how old you are. So skinwise, women who have a late menopause have a big advantage over those who lose their estrogen early. And so do women with a little extra weight, because their fat tissue continues to make a small amount of estrogen even after menopause.

Estrogen is not the fountain of youth, but it can definitely make a difference in the quality of your skin, so give some thought to hormone replacement therapy after menopause if there's no reason you can't use it. Although it can't change the effects of genetic aging or overexposure to the sun, it can help hold off the changes that are specifically due to estrogen loss and can improve your skin by adding fat, moisture, and collagen.

Women on HRT tend to look younger than their years, with thicker, moister, more flexible skin. Research has found, for example, that skin is only half as thick in women nearing 60 who do not take estrogen as it is among those who do.

THE EXTRINSIC FACTORS

Neither of the above culprits has anywhere near the destructive effect on skin as does overexposure to the sun's ultraviolet rays. An estimated 80 percent of all visible signs of aging and 90 percent of skin cancers are caused by the sun.

Although the results of sun damage usually don't become obvious until many years after it occurs—the wrinkles you see today had their genesis in your teens—sunlight accelerates the processes of chronological aging.

Too much sun can be harmful in another way, too. It can impair the skin's immune response, weakening its ability to destroy invading bacteria and viruses and promoting DNA damage that increases the risk of skin cancer.

Other environmental assaults on the surface of your body can add to the damage. These include smoking, extreme temperatures, wind, dry air, air pollution, and prolonged exposure to direct heat such as heating pads and open fires.

Smoker's Skin

Your skin is three times more likely to wrinkle early if you smoke than if you don't, according to several studies. Smoking contributes to lines around your eyes and mouth and, worse, constricts the small blood vessels of your face, reducing the supply of oxygen to the delicate facial tissues. Never mind that it also stains your teeth.

What's more, both smoking and ultraviolet light increase the production of free radicals that damage cells, inhibit DNA repair, and promote aging.

WHAT YOU CAN DO *NOW*

Stay out of the sun. Sun protection is by far the top wrinkle preventer, so avoid the sun if you can and use sunscreen and sunblock if you can't. Sun is the skin's arch enemy, not only encouraging structural damage and wrinkles but cancer as well. It hastens the aging process by destroying collagen and elastin, the key components of the dermis, the layer beneath the epidermis that gives skin its strength and elasticity.

A suntan, which you probably think makes you look healthier, is actually a superficial indicator of the cellular damage caused by prolonged sun exposure. It is your body's response to injury and an effort to prevent more harm from the sun's burning rays by increasing its pigment. Its effect won't show up for maybe ten or twenty years, but the more sun you've had, the older your skin will eventually look, feel, and behave.

If you have already spent years lying in the sun, developing a deep dark tan every year, there's nothing you can do now except stop doing it. But like smoking, it always pays to quit sunning because it's the only way to put an end to the self-destruction and give your tissues time to accomplish a certain degree of recuperation.

Meanwhile, follow these rules:

1. Don't step out of the house without first applying a sunblock or a broad-spectrum sunscreen with an SPF (sun protector factor) of at least 15. Sunblocks such as titanium dioxide and zinc oxide physically block or reflect both UVA and UVB rays, while sunscreens are chemicals that form a film over the skin and absorb the ultraviolet radiation.

   An SPF rating measures only a sunscreen's ability to block UVB, the rays that burn. SPF 15 means it will take your skin fifteen times longer to burn than it does with no protection. Most sunscreens absorb only UVB, the primary culprit in causing visible damage such as redness and sunburn, but are transparent to UVA, the nonburning rays that penetrate deeper, can pass through glass, and are suspected of being even more damaging and carcinogenic than UVB.

   A new study on mice at the M.D. Anderson Cancer Center in Houston has raised questions about whether sunscreens can protect against melanoma, the deadliest of all skin cancers, and, in fact, may even encourage more cases of it. That's because the usual sunscreens, by allowing you to remain much longer in the sun without burning, may encourage prolonged exposure to the more dangerous UVA.

So our advice to you is to use a sunscreen lotion that contains the chemical compound Parsol 1789 (avobenzone), the only ingredient that has been approved by the FDA specifically for UVA protection, giving you broad-spectrum protection against both UVB and UVA.

UVA and UVB

Ultraviolet light includes ultraviolet B (UVB), which is responsible for the production of vitamin D in the skin and the tanning and burning effects of the sun, and ultraviolet A (UVA), which has been implicated in causing skin cancer and cataracts.

---

2. Apply the sunscreen liberally at least a half hour before you expose yourself, and reapply it every two or three hours. Use it more often if you swim or sweat heavily, even if it is labeled "waterproof."
3. Replace your sunscreens after two years, as they may deteriorate and lose their protective abilities.
4. Wear sunglasses, long sleeves, long pants, and a brimmed hat when possible. Don't count on wet clothes or loose weaves for protection.
5. Remember that the sun is especially dangerous between 10 A.M. and 3 P.M. Try to limit your exposure to other times of the day. You are no safer when the sky is cloudy because the rays not only penetrate the clouds but also reflect off their edges.
6. Remember that ultraviolet radiation is reflected and intensified by sand, water, snow, buildings, and sidewalks. And that your exposure is greater at higher altitudes and, of course, the closer your proximity to the equator. The UV rays even penetrate several feet underwater.
7. Don't count on red skin to alert you to sun damage.

As you get older, you sunburn less easily because your inflammatory response diminishes over time. Besides, damage from UVA rays doesn't show up as a burn.

Beware of Drug Interaction

Some commonly used drugs raise your chances of getting sunburned by increasing the skin's sensitivity to ultraviolet light. Among the photosensitive drugs are some antibiotics such as tetracycline; tretinoin (Retin-A); nonsteroidal anti-inflammatory drugs; some sleeping pills; and diuretics. Check the labels of the drugs you take. If they mention sun sensitivity as a possible side effect, be especially careful to stay out of the sun's way.

"I am in my late fifties and I don't seem to get as sunburned as I once did, even when I'm out in the sun the same length of time. Does that means I am safe now?"

Definitely not. You just don't burn as easily anymore. But you're racking up more sun damage than ever, despite the lack of an early warning signal, because your skin is thinner now. That permits more radiation to reach the layers vulnerable to cancer and aging.

"I don't tan easily anymore, although I spend just as much time as ever outside. Is that normal?"

Yes, because your protective pigment cells are fewer and less active than they were when you were young. But, again, that doesn't mean the sun's ultraviolet rays are not inflicting their customary destruction. In fact, they can be even more damaging.

"What about tanning parlors? Are they any safer than sitting in the sun?"

No, although their predominant type of UV radiation is UVA, the tanning rays that are much less likely to cause a burn. However, most tanning beds emit UVA at an intensity even greater than that of natural sunlight and these deep penetrating rays are thought to be even more destructive and carcinogenic than UVB.

"Aren't you more protected once you've got a nice tan?"

Yes, but you have damaged your skin in achieving your tan. A tan is a response to injury.

"Does self-tanning cream protect your skin?"

No. It's just a dye that colors your skin.

"What about vitamin D? Isn't sunlight needed to get your quota of it?"

The sun converts inactive vitamin D to an active form that the body can use, but fifteen minutes of sun a day is plenty in moderate latitudes. Besides, milk is fortified with vitamin D and is a safer source.

DRY SKIN: WHAT TO DO ABOUT IT

Keep in mind that you are now suffering from a chronic condition. Your epidermal cells don't hold as much moisture as they once did, and they don't renew themselves anywhere near as quickly. The cells pile up, stick together, and become progressively dehydrated. All of this means you have dry skin that looks flaky or powdery, feels rough, and may get very itchy especially in the winter. Here's what you can do:

Moisturize and Lubricate   In most cases, the solution is simple: massive lubrication. Although moisturizers don't add water to the structure of the skin, they reduce the loss of water from its surface by sealing it in. If your skin is dry, use one every day, applying it just after a bath or a wash when the skin is damp. Use one containing sunscreen if you're going out in the sun.

Grease up regularly at night, again when the skin has been hydrated, using an oil-based cream or ointment, petroleum jelly, mineral or vegetable oil, baby oil, vegetable shortening, or something fancier if you like. The greasier the better. Many dermatologists say that, although it's messy, petroleum jelly is the best choice of all, followed by lanolin. As for commercial lubricants that are a combination of oil and water, the creams are more effective than the lotions because they contain more oil.

Hydrate Your Body from Within   Drink plenty of liquids. Try for eight 8-ounce glasses of fluids, preferably water, a day. Avoid dehydrators such as alcohol, caffeine, diuretics, dry air, and saunas.

Don't Be Obsessively Clean   Wash your skin as little as possible. Hot water and soap tend to damage cell membranes and make the skin more permeable. When you shower, use tepid water and skip the soap when you can, especially soap that's perfumed. If you must wash more, use a soap substitute like Cetaphil, SFC, or Moisturel. Soap breaks down the natural oil barrier that lubricates the skin and can do more damage than good. Don't take long hot baths and stay out of hot tubs.

Humidify   A humidifier (clean it every day and add a drop of bleach for each quart of water in the vaporizer reservoir to prevent fungal growth that can promote allergy), a lot of house plants, and a pot of water on the radiator can add moisture to the air. Hot steam vaporizers and self-sterilizing models do not require maintenance to prevent fungal growth.

Drinker's Skin

Excessive elbow-bending is hazardous to your skin, according to the American Academy of Facial Plastic and Reconstructive Surgery. It dehydrates it by drawing water away from its surface, increases the problem of broken capillaries, causes blood vessels to dilate, and gives you an unattractive "alcohol glow."

OILY SKIN: SOME WOMEN'S PROBLEM

Oddly enough, some women's skin gets oilier (although perhaps drier on the surface) as they get older, sometimes leading to adult acne for the first time in their lives. This happens when the male hormones, or androgens, that women produce along with the female variety become more influential because of the drop in estrogen production, especially if you are particularly sensitive to it. The androgens stimulate the oil glands (and perhaps facial hair, too).

If that's the case with you, skip all the grease suggested above and treat your skin as if you were an oily-skinned teenager again. Wash it frequently and use a non-oily moisturizer (glycerine and water) to prevent water loss.

If you develop acne or acne rosacea, fairly common after the age of 40, make an appointment with a dermatologist, who will prescribe the proper medication.

Caution: If your skin goes through an abrupt change from

dry to oily, especially if it is accompanied by facial hair and acne, promptly report it to your doctor as this may indicate a significant underlying condition.

WRESTLING WITH WRINKLES

Wrinkles, one of the most unwelcome manifestations of advancing years, can be blamed mostly on too much time spent basking in the sun. Other villains include smoking, chronological aging, rapid weight loss, gravity, and a lack of estrogen circulating in your body. Some you can do something about, others you can't.

Wrinkles—eventually—are inevitable. You can't escape them. But you can forestall them and minimize them by starting right now to protect your skin from more sun damage. In fact, you can do nothing better for your skin than staying out of the sun. Once you stop instigating more damage, the skin can reconstitute itself to a remarkable degree.

You can also help restore your skin by taking estrogen replacement after menopause, if it is right for you, because this hormone plays an important part in keeping the skin thick, moist, and flexible. Topical treatments are another route to a less wrinkled epidermis.

RETIN-A

Studies have shown that regular use of tretinoin or retinoic acid (a vitamin A derivative marketed as Retin-A) can minimize some of the superficial wrinkles of sun-damaged skin. The results of a large study suggest that after four to six months' treatment, there are subtle changes in the skin including less fine wrinkling, fewer liver spots, thicker epidermis, and fewer abnormalities.

Retin-A, available only by prescription, smoothes the outermost layer of skin by exfoliating it. In other words, it removes the dead cells cluttering the surface of aging skin and encourages faster proliferation of new cells. It also thickens the epidermis, the next layer, somewhat and irritates the skin slightly, bringing more blood flow to the surface.

What Retin-A won't do is erase deep wrinkles or tighten drooping skin. And it has its side effects. Many users at least initially experience skin peeling or irritation, and all become more susceptible to sun damage, so a sunscreen must be used daily. Most important, the beneficial effects gradually fade when the drug is discontinued.

If you decide to try Retin-A, start with the lowest concentration to minimize the chance of adverse reactions, which may include red dry skin or a rash. Apply it in the evening to reduce the sun-sensitizing effect.

ALPHA-HYDROXY ACIDS (AHAs)

These substances are the latest weapon in the war against wrinkles caused by aging and the sun. The same natural acids found in fruits, sugarcane, and sour milk that have been used for years by dermatologists, they have been rediscovered and refined. The accomplishments of the AHAs are similar to those of Retin-A—improved skin texture, reduced fine lines, and lightened brown spots—but they are thought to work by loosening the bonds holding skin cells of the uppermost layer, hastening the normal shedding of excess dead cells. And, the theory goes, they thicken the living cell layer of the epidermis and boost the skin's ability to retain water.

The alpha-hydroxy acids include glycolic acid (from sugarcane); lactic acid (from sour milk); malic acid (from apples); citric acid (citrus fruits); tartaric acid (grapes), and a few semisynthetic compounds.

The advantages of the AHAs over Retin-A are that the acids don't make you supersensitive to the sun, aren't as irritating, and are relatively inexpensive. Carelessly used in strong concentrations, however, they can cause injury and scarring. Here, too, the results fade when you stop using them.

Now incorporated into many upscale skin-care products but in very low and therefore not very effective concentrations, the alpha-hydroxy acids work best in higher concentrations that require a prescription or as skin peels performed in skin-care salons or the dermatologist's office.

"What other treatments are available for getting rid of wrinkles and lines?"

Only the more aggressive procedures performed by dermatologists or plastic surgeons. *Chemical peels* use an acid solution to destroy the outer layer of skin, exposing the new skin underneath. Treatments range from superficial to mild to deep, and can erase wrinkles and lines.

Dermabrasion, another technique for removing surface layers of skin, erasing lines and scars, and revealing fresh new skin, mechanically sands off the top layer.

Soft-tissue augmentation involves injecting the skin with fillers to plump up wrinkles and lines and fill pitted scars. The most widely used filler today is collagen for filling in hollows. It lasts a few months before you need a new treatment. Some dermatologists are now using fat injections as well, filling deep hollows and plumping up loose skin with fat taken from your own body. These, too, last only a short time. Silicone injections for this purpose are now outlawed, despite the fact that silicone has been used to coat the inside of syringes for the last thirty-five years.

And, of course, *cosmetic plastic surgery* can counter the effects of gravity and age by redraping the skin, removing wrinkles and sagging skin.

Sources of Information

For information about procedures and referrals to board-certified dermatologic surgeons who perform skin treatments in your state, call the American Society for Dermatologic Surgery's hotline, 800-441-2737. Or contact the American Academy of Dermatology, 930 N. Meacham Road, Schaumburg, Illinois 60173-4965; 708-330-0230.

You can get information and referrals for board-certified plastic surgeons from the Plastic Surgery Information Service, 800-635-0635.

"Can you exfoliate your skin yourself with a washcloth or a brush?"

Definitely, if you take your own skin type into consideration. Anything that exfoliates, from loofahs, to brushes, or even a sturdy washcloth, can help get rid of dead skin. Take it easy, however. Injury is not the objective.

"My skin has been very itchy and easily irritated in the last few years. The doctor says I have dermatitis and there's nothing to do about it except use moisturizers and lubricants. What causes it?"

Very common as you get older, dermatitis in most cases is simply very dry skin, most noticeable in the winter when the heat is on and the humidity is low. Follow the advice above. It can also be caused by chemicals in soap or cleaning agents. Or it may be an allergy.

"I've developed rosacea on my face in the last couple of years. I never had it before and I am wondering if it was caused by menopause. What can I do about it?"

Rosacea is an acnelike condition characterized by flushing or redness on the cheeks, nose, chin, or forehead, bloodshot eyes, little pustules, and dilated blood vessels. It is not caused by menopause but it's not uncommon for women to develop it around that time. Rosacea has to be treated or it tends to get worse, so get your doctor's advice on medical therapy and lifestyle changes. In general, avoid whatever triggers the flare-ups in your case. Some of the most common triggers are spicy or hot foods, sun, wind, cold, stress, and certain ingredients in cosmetics and skin-care products. For helpful information, contact the National Rosacea Society, 220 South Cook St., Barrington IL 60010 (708-382-5567).

"I feel chilly much more easily now in my sixties than I used to. Why is that?"

You feel colder because you *are* colder. With less subcutaneous fat, lower metabolism, and a decline in the activity of sweat glands, the skin becomes a less efficient regulator of body temperature. Besides, you probably don't exercise as much as you used to and so produce less body heat.

"I bruise very easily now, much more than I ever did before. Now all I have to do is bump against something and I've got a nasty-looking black-and-blue mark. What's the reason for that?"

Not only does your skin get thinner with every birthday but you have less protective cushioning because of the gradual loss of your subcutaneous fat layer that has always acted as a shock absorber. In addition, the walls of the blood vessels in your skin have become thinner and more fragile because of age and the decline in estrogen production. So those blood vessels break and bleed with less trauma than they used to.

A caution: Bruising can also be the symptom of a blood disorder or a side effect of certain medications such as aspirin and other anticoagulants, nonsteroidal anti-inflammatory drugs, and quinine. So it is worth mentioning to your physician.

"It takes much longer for my skin to heal now in my sixties than it did when I was younger. Is this normal?"

Yes. Because the mechanisms of healing, such as the formation of collagen and the development of new blood vessels, no longer work as well as they used to, cuts and other injuries may take longer to repair themselves.

"I have much less color in my skin than I did when I was younger and, in fact, it sometimes looks rather gray. What's the reason for that?"

As you age, blood circulation tends to decrease, resulting in less blood flow to the skin and rosiness to your cheeks.

Get Moving

Anything you do that helps your entire body will help your skin fight wrinkles. Vigorous exercise increases the blood supply to the skin, improving its overall health and giving you a rosier color. Sweating from exercise gets rid of metabolic wastes and cleanses the skin as well.

BUMPS, LUMPS, SPOTS, AND OTHER HAPPENINGS

A variety of skin changes—some of them benign, some not so benign, and most of them induced by longtime exposure to the sun—tend to make their first appearances in your forties or fifties. It is wise not to ignore them.

Aways check them out with your physician or a dermatologist if they have suddenly appeared; if they bleed or get crusty; if they change in shape, size, or color; or if they look strange in any way whatsoever. Even without such occurrences, it is wise to have your family doctor look your skin over during your regular checkups and to schedule a full head-to-toe skin examination with a dermatologist once a year, just to be sure all is well. You have reached the age when problems may emerge.

"What can be done about those 'liver spots' I've developed on the backs of my hands? Are they caused by nutritional deficiencies? Are they inevitable? Are they dangerous?"

Here's what we now know about all of the bumps, lumps, and spots that appear on the skin after age 40:

Liver Spots Lentigos, known as liver spots or age spots, have nothing to do with the liver. Nor are they connected with what you eat or don't eat. They are flat brown blotches of extra pigment that appear on your face and hands as you get older and they multiply with age. Essentially large freckles that result from lifelong exposure to the sun, most of them are harmless, although not easy to remove. (Again, if they are new and especially if they appear on your face, let a dermatologist make sure they are age spots and not early cancer.)

Commercial skin lighteners may eventually fade them slightly, or you might try hydroquinone, a skin-lightening drug in a lotion or cream, in a 2 percent concentration that's available only by prescription. Another seemingly effective way to treat them is with Retin-A (tretinoin). In a recent study, Retin-A faded facial age spots in 83 percent of those treated. During the next six months, spots that had disappeared did not return in those who stopped using the cream.

Alpha-hydroxy acids, especially glycolic acid, which has the smallest molecules of the group and therefore can penetrate more deeply, promise to deliver the same results, again used faithfully for at least several months. If you are going to do it yourself, use only a low concentration (12 percent is usually recommended, available by prescription) and leave the stronger preparations to the physicians who specialize in this treatment.

Liver spots can also be treated with chemical peels, electrodessication, cryosurgery (freezing), laser, or applications of topical trichlorocetic acid, all performed in the doctor's office. Once the spots are removed this way, they won't return, although of course new ones may appear.

Moles At last, something besides wine that improves with age! Moles, most of them benign tumors of the skin that may be brown or almost black or pink or tan, usually disappear over the years.

If, in the meantime, you develop a *new* mole or you notice that a mole you've had around for a long time has started to grow, change color, or look different in any way, waste no time scheduling an appointment with your doctor to be checked for skin cancer (see below).

Some precancerous moles and other such bumps have been found to improve with applications of Retin-A twice a day, as reported in a new study at the University of Pennsylvania.

Seborrheic Keratoses Waxy, slightly raised, sometimes crusty patches that look like they've been stuck on the skin—

usually on your forearms, legs, back, or even your abdomen—seborrheic keratoses are harmless although not pretty. Becoming more and more numerous as your birthdays roll by, they can vary in size from the head of a pin to bigger than a half-dollar. You can safely leave them alone as they won't turn malignant and they aren't contagious unless they become infected with a wart virus. On the other hand, a malignant melanoma may look like a seborrheic keratosis and vice versa. Since only your doctor will know for sure, schedule that yearly skin checkup.

It is not a good idea to scrape these waxy patches off with your fingernails because you may cause infections and even scarring. Besides, they may grow right back. Better to have them removed professionally. Or to eradicate them in their early stages with regular use of an AHA such as Lac-Hydrin.

A word of caution: If you develop dozens or hundreds of seborrheic keratoses within several months, see your doctor as they may be an indication of a much more serious disorder.

Actinic Keratoses Caused by overexposure to the sun, these little growths are usually found on exposed skin and especially among fair-skinned people. Actinic keratoses are rough, dry, and pinkish, and should be removed because they can be precancerous. Go to a dermatologist who can scrape them off, remove them with electric current, or freeze them off with liquid nitrogen. Remember that these scaly spots signify many years of sun damage. Use them as a reminder to schedule regular skin examinations and to stay out of the sun.

Spider Veins Tiny dilated red and blue blood vessels just under the skin, usually appearing on the thighs and ankles, spider veins are not a serious health problem, although they too are not beautiful. Probably the result of a genetic predisposition, spider veins can be made worse by pregnancy, obesity, trauma, and a lot of standing. Probably 90 percent of women have them after 30 and then they steadily intensify.

The usual treatment for spider veins is sclerotherapy, when a chemical solution is injected through fine needles into the veins. The solution irritates, scars, and seals off the veins, which eventually shrink and fade. Virtually painless, sclerotherapy is done in the doctor's office.

Stretch Marks   Although there is no cure for stretch marks, they do improve with time. By the way, the old folk remedies—including cocoa butter and vitamin E oil—won't do a thing for them.

Sebaceous Hyperplasia   These collections of whitish-yellow bumps that look like small doughnuts and are found mainly on the face are the results of time and hormonal changes. Your dermatologist can flatten them with an electric needle after making sure they are not something more serious.

Blotchy Pigmentation (Melasma)   Increased pigmentation, a slight darkening of the skin here and there, can be blamed on hormonal changes as well as overexposure to the sun. Although it is usually a young woman's problem that's often initiated by pregnancy, in older women it may be a side effect of oral contraceptives or high-dose estrogen replacement. It is rare at the usual HRT doses.

What can be done about the pigmented areas? Stop the oral contraceptives or the HRT if it is the cause of the problem. Or talk to your doctor about lowering the dose. Protect your skin from the sun with a UVA-UVB sunscreen. Try Retin-A or alpha-hydroxy acids. Or try hydroquinone, a bleaching cream, in no more than 2 percent concentration. In higher concentrations it has the potential of irritating and inflaming the skin, sometimes making your situation even worse.

In the doctor's office, you may have the pigmented areas frozen off with liquid nitrogen, removed by a skin peel, or dessicated by an electric needle. The more aggressive methods such as chemical skin peels, however, must be used with extreme caution.

SKIN CANCER

Now let's get down to more serious matters: skin conditions that are not so benign. Skin cancer is not only the most common form of cancer—an estimated one out of six Americans can now expect to get it in a lifetime—but it is becoming almost epidemic with more new cases diagnosed every year than all other types of cancer combined. It is also the most curable cancer when lesions are detected and removed in the early stages. So, obviously, it is essential to go to a specialist promptly if you notice any of its common characteristics.

Use of Retin-A has been found in a recent study to fade or even erase some moles that may grow into skin cancer, catching abnormal tissue before it becomes malignant. Ask your doctor whether any of your odd-looking bumps would profit from it.

SKIN CANCER: WHO'S AT HIGHEST RISK?

- Sun worshippers.
- Women. Women are four times more likely than men to get skin cancer.
- Fair-skinned, blue-eyed individuals with blond or red hair. Their skin, because it has the least amount of melanin or pigmentation cells, is the most vulnerable.
- Women who are middle aged or older. The risk steadily increases with age; the older you get, the lower

your capacity to repair DNA damaged by the sun, an ability directly related to your susceptibility to cancer.
- Affluent, highly educated people, perhaps because they are more likely to have spent many vacations at sun-drenched resorts.
- Those who have had previous skin cancer, especially basal cell and squamous cell cancer.

BASAL CELL CARCINOMA

The most common form of skin cancer, basal cell usually appears as single, small, pearly bumps with tiny blood vessels and rolled edges, sometimes doughnut-shaped. It grows slowly, may bleed and crust over, but never heals. The bumps are usually found on the face, neck, or hands—in other words, the parts of you that have been most exposed to the sun. This kind of cancer doesn't spread but it can cause serious local destruction.

SQUAMOUS CELL CARCINOMA

This is a firm nodule or a flat red patch with a scaly or crusty surface. It may ulcerate and it, too, never heals. It is typically found on the rim of the ear, face, back, upper chest, arms, legs, and other sun-exposed areas. Untreated, it can grow bigger and can eventually spread to other parts of the body, especially if it originates on mucus membranes such as the lips.

MALIGNANT MELANOMA

The deadliest form of skin cancer, melanoma is also the least common. Although it can spread quickly throughout the body, it is almost always completely curable in its early stages. It may appear anywhere on the body; women often get it on the legs, while the back is a more likely location for men. A melanoma may be small and deep or it may grow laterally over months or years. It usually looks like an asymmetrical dark or multicolored or speckled mole with an irregular ragged or blurred edge. See this kind of growth and run to your doctor.

Check Your Own Skin

Make a habit of examining your entire body, top to toe, back and front, in the mirror every month or so. Check your back and buttocks with a hand mirror. Don't forget the soles of your feet and between your toes, the back of your neck and your scalp.

CONCERNS ABOUT HAIR

Your skin, of course, is undoubtedly the biggest concern you have about your outer surface, but many women at this time in their lives notice changes in their hair growth, both on their heads and their bodies, and find their nails are giving them problems they never had before.

"Why is my hair getting thin on top? I've been forced to find new ways to arrange my hair so the thinning doesn't show."

All women gradually lose hair as they get older, but some lose enough to cause them real heartache. If your hair has become noticeably scantier, blame it on your genes with a little help from your hormones. Chronic androgenetic alopecia—hereditary hair loss—causes marked thinning in about 10 percent of women by the time they are 40. By 60, that figure jumps to about 40 percent, although only about one in five women has enough loss to cause a problem apparent to others.

FAST FACTS ABOUT HAIR LOSS

- Patterned androgenic hair loss is usually caused by a combination of hormonal factors, hereditary factors, and age.
- Women don't lose their hair as obviously as men do. They generally experience diffuse thinning over the entire scalp without developing obvious bald spots.
- Every hair follicle goes through a cycle. There is a growth phase, then a resting and a shedding phase. In hereditary hair loss, the growth phase becomes shorter and the resting phase longer.
- The healthy scalp loses about 100 hairs a day, normally replaced by a similar number of new ones. But as you get older, the number of hairs you replace diminishes because you are progressively losing hair follicles. If more hairs consistently fall out than grow back, you are losing ground.
- While all women produce some androgens (male hormones), some women tend to have hair follicles that are overly sensitive to them. This hormonal sensitivity often shows up after menopause when the androgens you produce become more influential because they are no longer adequately opposed by estrogen.
- A wide range of disorders, from fungal infections to lupus, and certain drugs can also cause temporary or permanent hair loss.

• A very rapid loss of hair over a few months sometimes signifies a serious illness, so check it out with your physician immediately.

WHAT YOU CAN DO *NOW*

Hereditary hair loss is a problem that has always defied the experts, and only recently has a drug come along that can help some women. To date, here's what we know:

Rogaine (minoxidil) is your best bet so far, although few women who use it have significant hair growth. Recently approved by the FDA for women, it is a prescription lotion that is applied to the scalp twice a day and works only as long as it is used. It has proved to stimulate some regrowth, or at least prevent further hair loss, in some people, although it will never give you back a luxurious head of hair.

Hormone replacement therapy won't restore your hair growth very much, but it may thicken it up a little. On the other hand, it can help to slow down the rate of loss by helping to balance out the effect of androgens on your follicles.

Aldactone (spironolactone), a diuretic with antiandrogenic properties that can block the growth of undesirable facial and body hair, sometimes encourages growth of hair on your head. It works only as long as you use it and has not yet been approved for this use by the FDA.

"The hair on my arms and legs has almost disappeared, I never have to shave under my arms anymore, and I have very little hair left in the pubic area. Is that all a normal part of the aging process?"

Yes. Body hair is under the control of your hormones. When you lose estrogen, this kind of hair usually goes with it.

"I'm losing hair on the top of my head and getting some on my face where I never had it before. Why is that happening and what can I do about it?"

After menopause, many women find hair growing on their face and/or body where it never grew before and where it certainly is not welcome, especially since the hair is often dark and coarse. That's because in some women the male hormones they normally produce in addition to estrogen become more dominant as the estrogen level drops off. When estrogen cannot block the action of these androgens at the hair follicle receptors, hair tends to grow in a more male pattern.

The best solution is to take estrogen replacement, which won't remove existing hairs but may stop new hairs from growing in the wrong places. If that's not in your cards, you can try other measures. One alternative is a drug that has not yet been approved for this use by the FDA, although it is approved as a diuretic. This is Aldactone (spironolactone), a receptor blocker for facial and body hair. It works for some women but only for as long as you use it.

The only permanent way to remove unwanted hair is by electrolysis, which destroys the hair root with an electric current. Expensive and tedious, this procedure should be performed by a trained and experienced electrologist. Temporary removal can be accomplished by shaving, tweezing, waxing, or depilitating. And some women prefer bleaching the hair so it isn't so obvious. If you decide to try this method, be aware that you may get a local reaction from the bleach and the skin may heal with hyperpigmentation.

CONCERNS ABOUT NAILS

Nails are not exempt from the aging process. What they do is become thinner, more brittle, and more bendable as time goes on. They also grow more slowly, tend to lose their "moons" and develop longitudinal ridges. (If you have developed thick irregular nails, however, the culprit may not be age but a fungal infection.)

Composed of a protein called keratin just like their cousins skin and hair, nails grow from deep inside the skin out of living tissues, although they themselves are dead tissue and nothing you can put on them will make them grow any better or any stronger. Calcium supplements don't help since nails are not bone. And forget gelatin. However, you might try Biotin—buy it at the health food store—in doses of 2 milligrams a day. It may reduce the brittleness, according to dermatologist Wendy Keller Epstein.

WHAT YOU CAN DO *NOW*

Here are some sensible things to remember about nails that are now more fragile than they used to be:

1. If they tend to break or split when you're cutting them, soak them first in warm water for about ten minutes. They are more resilient when moist. On the other hand, let them dry thoroughly before you file them. And keep them short.
2. Promptly file down any little nicks or splits before they turn into major breaks. Then use moisturizer on them.
3. Don't use nail hardeners. They dry nails out too much, encouraging breakage. Polish remover is also extremely drying, so use it as infrequently as possible.
4. Although you can add some strength by using a base coat, two coats of nail polish, and a top coat, it's better not to use polish at all. That's because you must remove it occasionally and the remover can do damage.
5. There's no known way to get rid of nail ridges, so simply buff them gently until smooth.
6. Moisturize your nails just as you do your skin and rub

petroleum jelly on them at night. Or soak them in water for five minutes, then apply an alpha-hydroxy acid moisturizer. If you can stand sleeping in cotton gloves over the moisturized or greased nails, all the better.

7. Since your fingernails aren't all that strong anymore, quit using them as handy tools.

8. Protect your nails from the ravages of water, chemicals, and detergents by wearing rubber gloves. Nails are highly permeable. Water causes them to swell and then shrink when they dry out. Chemicals and detergents dry them out too. Too much of these and they're more brittle than ever.

"Can I get AIDS from a manicure?"

That's very doubtful since the HIV virus doesn't last in air and certainly not in alcohol or disinfectants. However, other viruses such as the hepatitis virus are not susceptible to disinfectants. Therefore, we'd advise you to take your own cutting tools along when you get a professional manicure.

Chapter 19

YOUR FIGURE: STAYING IN SHAPE AS TIME GOES BY

YOU'VE PUT ON A FEW EXTRA POUNDS in the last couple of years and find them almost impossible to take off. You've definitely developed a bit of a potbelly. Your rib cage has expanded and so has your pelvis. Your clothes don't fit as well as they used to and, even if your weight hasn't changed very much, your waistline certainly has and you can't get into the size you've worn for many years. You're eating the same as you always have. What's going on here?

What's going on is that your body is changing. Blame it mostly on your metabolism that, after about 40, slows down as your birthdays go by and requires fewer calories to sustain your customary body weight. Keep eating the same amount of food and the pounds will accumulate. A woman who could eat 2,000 calories a day in adolescence has to scale back to about 1,200 a day by age 65. If you are typical, you'll put on ten to fifteen pounds in the midlife decades, most of them around the middle. You'll acquire the most pounds between the ages of 40 and 50, with a noticeable upward spurt in the first couple of years after menopause. Unless you make some changes in your daily habits, you'll put on a little more each year as you edge into your fifties and sixties, before you level off at around 65.

Again if you are typical, the configuration of your body—the distribution of weight on your frame—begins to change now too, so you'll end up with a figure that's not quite the same as the one you started out with. Hips and breasts tend to lose some of their fat tissue and, with it, their firmness, while fat piles up on waist, abdomen, shoulders, and upper back.

Responsible, along with the metabolic slowdown, for much of these changes is the loss of lean muscle mass. By the age of 70, you're likely to have a third fewer muscle cells than you had at 20. And as you lose muscle, you gain more fat, a combination that slows down your metabolism because muscle burns calories at a much faster rate than fat.

You also lose height with the years. At 40, maybe you're a half an inch or so shorter than you used to be; at 50, perhaps you've shrunk an inch; and in the next few decades you may lose up to two or three inches, maybe even four inches if you have osteoporosis. You're shrinking because of compression of the spinal column, the result of general wear and tear and a gradual loss of bone mass (see Chapter 4).

With spinal compression comes an expanded rib cage and a bigger waistline because you are now packing more contents into less space.

FAST FACTS ABOUT WEIGHT

- Weight is a key factor in your health and becomes more and more important as you get older. The "ideal" weights widely published by insurance companies years ago are too low for most people over 40. Many studies have concluded that you live longer if you put on a few, but only a few, ·pounds as you get older and then stay stable. Losing your excess pounds can lower the risk of developing many diseases, including diabetes, arthritis, coronary heart disease, and cancer. In fact, a loss of just ten or fifteen pounds is often all that is needed to counter the most serious adverse health effects of obesity.

- Your body type and weight have been determined primarily by your genes. You must work very hard—especially now—if you insist on making changes in that biological heritage. People come in assorted inherited shapes and sizes. Some women are naturally thin and elongated while others have an equally natural tendency to be heavier and stockier, a tendency that is accentuated as they get older.

- Fat distribution alters with the seasons, say Tufts Medical School researchers who studied healthy post-menopausal women. At the same weights, the women were leaner all over in warm months, fatter in cold, especially in their midsections and legs.

- Pear-shaped women—those who carry most of their fat on their hips and thighs—have been found to live longer than women who are shaped like apples, bigger in the waist than the hips.

- Smokers are likely to have more upper-body fat. This is the kind that's associated with health problems, although smokers are usually thinner overall than non-smokers.

- Multiple weight losses and gains are associated with shorter life spans. The lowest death rates are among those who maintain a fairly low and stable weight.

WHAT YOU CAN DO *NOW*

You can fight back! You can't prevent all of the normal body changes that come with age, but you can certainly minimize them by making some fairly simple changes in your daily routine. For motivation, keep in mind that you are now looking at your best opportunity to preserve your shape as well as your health. For perspective, remember that body changes are a natural phenomenon at this time in your life just as they were in adolescence and young adulthood, so quit blaming yourself for them. They haven't happened because of what you did or didn't do. Maybe your measurements aren't the same as they were at the senior prom, but neither are Elizabeth Taylor's or even Jane Fonda's.

Here are the steps you can take to keep these normal readjustments under control:

1. *Start preserving your bone structure.* The sturdier your bones are before menopause and the stronger they remain after that, the less vulnerable they will be for the rest of your life. You will shrink less, maintain your current figure more. Consume plenty of calcium, stop smoking, get a sufficient amount of weight-bearing exercise, and, unless there's very good reason for you to avoid it, start taking HRT after menopause; see Chapter 4.

2. *Keep your weight under control.* Not by counting calories, but by switching to a diet that includes fewer fats and more fruits, vegetables, and complex carbohydrates. Eating wisely has never been more important than it is in the middle years.

3. *Begin a regime of regular exercise.* Nothing fancy, but with aerobic and weight-training components to build up your lean-muscle mass and raise your metabolic rate, helping you burn calories, control your weight, and keep your fat deposits where they belong.

FIGHTING FAT: THE RECIPE

Simply cutting calories—going on a diet—to lose weight rarely works in the long term because it requires so much effort that you can't keep it up forever. You may lose some pounds initially, but you are almost sure to gain them right back again, not only because you revert to your old habits but because the body has a remarkable resistance to major weight change.

Besides, it is hazardous to your health to lose and gain weight time and time again. So your goal should be to maintain a relatively lean and steady weight. We all know that obesity (you are considered overweight if you're 20 percent above the "normal" weight for your body structure and obese at 30 percent) increases the risks of many diseases. But going to the other extreme, unless you were born with a naturally reedy body, is not realistic. Studies have recently strengthened the case for modest weight gain with age, and 10 percent over "ideal" is certainly not unhealthy when you are over 40. Settle for a weight that's comfortable, looks good, functions well, and can be maintained without enormous difficulty.

The easiest way to achieve a reasonable weight that you can maintain without constant torment is to make a permanent commitment to a sensible eating plan combined with regular exercise to raise the metabolic rate and build up lean muscle mass.

PART I: DIET

You don't need another "diet." You've seen hundreds of them and, if they worked, you wouldn't need help now. Forget diets and focus on making some simple changes in the kinds of foods you eat. Then your weight will take care of itself.

The key is low-fat eating. That means switching from typical fat-loaded foods to foods that contain a much lower level of fat and an increased amount of carbohydrates, most of them in the form of fruits and vegetables. Overweight is the result, not of the number of calories you consume, but of the percentage of fat you take in.

Despite what you learned in school ("a calorie is a calorie"), all calories are not created equal. Calorie for calorie, fat is by far the most fattening nutrient because it is more likely to become body fat than the same number of calories from carbohydrates. It is even possible to consume as many calories as you did before—if they are not from fat—and lose weight.

So, forget dieting. Instead, focus on adopting a healthy lifestyle. Eat as little fat as possible and fill up with fiber-rich fruits, vegetables, and starchy foods. Because fat has twice as many calories per ounce as either carbohydrates or protein, you will automatically reduce your caloric consumption without feeling unsatisfied. And you will find yourself losing weight without having to eat less.

Unless you've spent the last few years on Jupiter, you know how to do that: switch to low- or nonfat dairy foods, dressings and snacks, trim the fat off meat and poultry, ease up on the portions and frequency of fatty foods, and use as little fat as possible in food preparation and at the table. (By the way, fat is fat, animal or vegetable, so avoid *both* margarine and butter.) Not only will your weight improve on such a diet but so will your overall health. A low-fat diet must be the one you live by, except maybe on Thanksgiving or your birthday. It means that you don't have to continually focus on what you are eating or not eating. All you must think about is avoiding fat.

If you need help, join a weight-loss club. If you don't, pick an eating regime you can stick with. It doesn't matter how you arrange it—a big breakfast, a little breakfast, a big lunch and no dinner, whatever—as long as you keep the fat content down. To lose weight, go for a limit of less than 30 grams of fat per day. To maintain weight, stay under 35 grams.

PART II: EXERCISE

Exercise, the wonder drug of the nineties, provides the best single strategy for a long healthy life because it can improve your health, your shape, your sense of well-being, and even your life expectancy. Evidence is rapidly accumulating to show it protects against disease and death from ailments ranging from cardiovascular disease and osteoporosis to colon cancer and diabetes. It also increases your strength, raises your metabolism, replaces fat tissue with muscle mass, and burns up calories. Aside from the risk of injury, there's no downside to exercise, and it can do you an amazing amount of good.

But today, when few of us milk the cows every day at dawn, walk two miles to school and two miles back, or spend time scrubbing the floors and running after the chickens, it requires planning and a certain amount of determination to fit enough exertion into our lives. That means finding a form (or several forms) of exercise that work for you—physical activities that you don't loathe, may even enjoy, and can stick with week after week.

Although all by itself exercise is not very efficient at taking off weight, it can make the difference between success and failure when accompanied by a sensible eating plan. Working out burns calories and increases the ratio of muscle to body fat, which in turn speeds up metabolism so the body burns more calories even at rest.

Exercise *Now*

Because most women gain at least ten or fifteen pounds in their middle years, start preventing it before it happens or soon thereafter. Beginning at least two or three years before menopause, but ideally earlier, get started on a regular exercise and weight-training program to counter the increase in fat tissue and encourage the buildup of lean muscle mass.

GOOD REASONS TO GET A MOVE ON

The older you get, the more exercise you need to keep your metabolism humming along quickly enough to burn off calories and protect you from the diseases that become more common with age. Since you are now making less muscle and more fat, the only way for your system to be more efficient is to prime it with physical activity. If that's not enough to motivate you, consider the following:

Every Little Bit Helps. Even very mild exercise—just walking another block or two, climbing a flight of stairs, raking leaves in your yard—can help bring elevated blood pressure down to normal. And the latest evidence indicates that you can get benefit from exercise even when it's accomplished in short takes.

Thinner at the Same Weight. Even if exercise doesn't take off pounds, it can help you lose inches. A pound of muscle is more compact than a pound of fat.

Longer-Lasting Results. The people most likely to maintain weight losses are those who use physical exercise to lose weight and then continue to exercise regularly afterwards.

Heightened Resistance. According to a study by an exercise physiologist at the University of North Carolina, women who walk forty-five minutes a day are half as likely as their sedentary counterparts to get colds or the flu.

Lowered Cholesterol. In a three-year study at the University of Pittsburgh, researchers found that middle-aged women who increased their physical activity not only had the smallest increases in weight but also the biggest improvement in HDL cholesterol levels.

Never Too Late. It's never too late to become physically fit, despite years of sedentary living. Exercise can improve cardiovascular fitness, respiratory capacity, and strength at any age.

Mood Medicine. People who exercise regularly have been shown to be less depressed than couch potatoes.

Brain Medicine. Exercise increases oxygen and sugar available to the brain, helping it function better. It also helps offset the loss of capillary production later in life, giving the brain an increased blood supply. Researchers at the University of Kentucky found that adults tested at least 15 percent smarter after two weeks of an aerobic exercise program and scored even higher when tested months later.

Better Insulin Efficiency. Exercisers develop adult-onset diabetes about 40 percent less than nonexercisers.

Longer Life. Men who expend 2,000 calories a week in aerobic activity were found to add 2.5 years to their life expectancy. For women too, building muscle may be the best single strategy for a longer healthier life.

"Regular" Habits. Exercise tends to speed waste through the intestines, helping to regulate bowel movements and, probably for the same reason, reduce the chances of developing colon cancer.

Bone Savers. Regular weight-bearing exercise—such as weight lifting, jogging, dancing, or walking—can strengthen your bones and help ward off osteoporosis. Active women in their forties and fifties have been shown to have significantly greater bone density in their vertebrae and forearms than their sedentary peers.

WHAT TO DO

Aerobic Exercise Try moderately vigorous walking, jogging, swimming, biking, dancing, singles tennis—whatever gets your heart racing and your lungs working reasonably hard. Exercise at a rate at which you are aware of breathing hard but not so hard that you can't carry on a conversation. Aim for twenty to thirty minutes three to five times a week.

Exercise Equivalents

1 mile of walking = 1 mile of running = 3 miles of biking = 300 yards of swimming = 15 minutes of aerobics

---

Weight Training Work out with weights or resistance machines to build more muscle tissue. Start slowly and eventually strengthen all of the major muscle groups of the body. Exercise at least twenty minutes, at least three times a week. Be aware that 50 percent of a muscle's gain from exercise is lost in only seventy-two hours of inactivity!

No need to join an expensive gym unless you want to. Light hand weights plus pushups and situps are just as effective.

How to Begin an Exercise Program

- Choose one or more lifetime exercises that you really enjoy—or at least don't hate—so you'll be able to stick with them forever. For women who haven't led an athletic life, the best choice is walking. Everybody can do it; it's cheap, easy, and always available. You don't need equipment, special clothes (except for a good pair of comfortable shoes), a team, or even a partner.

- If you don't want to stay with the same old routine every day, alternate your activities. Every day choose from among several forms of exercise: walking, swimming, tennis, biking, working out, aerobics, climbing stairs. Indoors, outdoors, morning, noontime, evening. Whatever moves you.

- If you are self-motivated, exercise on your own. If you are not, hire a personal trainer, join a class or an exercise club, or make a date a few mornings a week with a couple of friends who also want to get fit.

- Get your doctor's approval first, and start slowly. If you've been sedentary for a while, begin modestly and gradually build to longer, harder, faster workouts over several weeks. The duration and intensity of your exercise can be safely increased at no more than 10 percent a week. Think of your program as a lifetime change to increased activity.

- Dress comfortably in roomy clothes, well-fitting supportive athletic shoes. Exercise indoors when it is very hot or cold outside. Drink plenty of water before, during, and after a workout.

- And don't overdo it. Rest whenever it seems necessary. You've got your whole life to stay fit; injuries are unnecessary time-outs. There is no finish line; it's the journey not the destination that counts.

- If your session leaves you feeling exhausted or in pain five minutes after you stop, you did more than you should. Cut back next time. If, however, you are comfortable after the same five minutes, stay at that level for a week and increase the periods of intense exercise by 10 percent each week.
- If you have been inactive for more than six weeks, consider yourself deconditioned and start exercising at a low intensity so that for the first five minutes you are not aware of breathing hard. Then continue a faster pace for two minutes, before slowing down again for a five-minute cooldown.
- Be consistent. To pay off in health gains and weight loss, any activity must be done at least three or four days a week for a minimum of twenty minutes each day.

Try this exercise regime:

MONDAY	Take a brisk walk
TUESDAY	Ride your bicycle or exercycle
WEDNESDAY	Swim at a moderate pace
THURSDAY	Take the day off
FRIDAY	Play a few sets of singles tennis
SATURDAY	Take a brisk walk
SUNDAY	Take the day off

Chapter 20

MOSTLY FEMALE: HEALTH PROBLEMS THAT AFFECT WOMEN MOST

MANY AILMENTS and conditions are much more common among women than men, sometimes because of hormonal differences, sometimes not. Here are the answers to some of the questions physicians hear over and over from their over-40 female patients.

"Why do women get varicose veins and men don't? Do varicose veins get worse as time goes on? My mother and my three aunts have them and now I'm getting them."

Men get varicose veins too, but not anywhere near as often as women, all of whom have them to one degree or another after age 30 or 35. Nobody knows exactly what causes them, but we do know the tendency is inherited, may have a hormonal basis, and is often exacerbated by pregnancy because of increased pelvic vein pressure.

Varicose veins are more of an unattractive nuisance than a serious health hazard, although they can cause considerable discomfort. They are surface veins whose valves have failed. All veins have valves that keep blood moving along toward the heart from the lower body and prevent it from backing up, much like the locks in a canal.

Since veins do not have muscular walls like arteries, they depend on the leg muscles to compress them and push the blood upward. When they are intact, the valves prevent back flow resulting from the force of gravity. When they fail, the blood backs up and pools, stretching the walls of the veins. Unfortunately, varicose veins do tend to get worse as you get older because the valves relax even more over time, extending the problem into other veins.

"Is there anything I can do to prevent my varicose veins from getting worse?"

The best preventive is exercise—walking, swimming, or biking, for example—that works the leg muscles and compresses the veins. Don't sit or stand around too much and, if you must, get up and walk around frequently or prop your feet on a foot stool. At every opportunity during the day, elevate your legs at least 90 degrees for half an hour or so.

Other suggestions: control your weight, avoid heavy lifting, and quit smoking. Don't cross your legs. Don't wear garters or knee-highs with tight bands that act like tourniquets, impeding free blood flow and increasing pressure on the valves.

Try wearing support stockings or support panty hose, which have changed a lot in the last few years and no longer look like bandages. They come in graduated pressures. Their purpose is to compress the legs to keep blood from accumulating in the veins when you stand.

"I'd like to have my varicose veins removed. What's the usual procedure?"

There are two: sclerotherapy and surgery. Sclerotherapy is an office procedure used mainly for small surface veins. It involves the injection of a chemical solution that irritates, scars, and seals the veins off so they fade away in a few weeks.

Surgical "stripping," performed under anesthesia in the hospital, is usually the preferred treatment because it has a far better cure rate. It removes the offending veins through a series of small incisions. You'll never miss them because there is a vast surrounding network of other veins that will expand and take over the job of sending blood back up to the heart.

"How does hormone replacement therapy affect varicose veins? I've heard you shouldn't take it if you have them."

For many years, it was thought that HRT might make varicose veins worse because high doses of estrogen can increase the clotting tendency. However, the tiny amount given in HRT is most unlikely to affect clotting and, besides, these swollen veins come not from a clotting problem but from leaky valves.

"Then why did my doctor recommend going off HRT after I had phlebitis?"

Phlebitis and thrombophlebitis are an entirely different problem than varicose veins. They are inflammatory conditions in veins deep inside the legs caused by an abnormal blood condition that affects the clotting mechanism. If you have a tendency to form clots in those deep veins, most doctors will take you off HRT because of the possibility that even its tiny dose of estrogen will exacerbate the problem.

"I've never had headaches, but since menopause I've been getting terrible migraines. Why?"

Migraines, which afflict women three times more than men, are often associated with falling estrogen levels—or at least a sudden change from high levels to low—which is why many younger women get them around the time of menstruation. Most of the time, the headaches improve with age and frequently vanish around the time of menopause. For some unfortunate women, however, they get worse. And for others, this is the time when they make their debut.

"Does hormone replacement make headaches better or worse?"

Sometimes better, sometimes worse. If your migraines seem to be related to HRT, talk to your gynecologist about trying one or more of the following:

- Take a smaller dose of estrogen to see if that helps.
- Change the type of estrogen you take from conjugated estrogen to pure estradiol or pure estrone.
- If you are on cyclical HRT (three weeks on, one week off) and get your headaches during your week off, start taking your estrogen every day of the month.
- Add a tiny dose of testosterone to your estrogen.

"Is it true that women have more gallbladder disease than men? If so, what's the reason?"

The gallbladder is a small sac tucked under the liver. Its main job is to store bile, a substance produced by the liver, and to release it into the small intestine through the bile duct to help the body digest fat. Gallstones form when cholesterol crystallizes around tiny particles in the gallbladder.

Gallbladder disease is at least twice as common in women than in men and typically occurs in those who are over 40, overweight, and have had more than one pregnancy. The reason is that estrogen, in its excretion through the liver, tends to concentrate the cholesterol in the bile, encouraging the formation of stones that then may get stuck in the bile duct. Women naturally make estrogen, overweight women make even more estrogen, and pregnant women produce over 1,000 times more estrogen than they did before.

Other factors that help to concentrate the bile include a

high consumption of dairy products and animal fats, very-low-calorie dieting with rapid weight loss, and low-fiber intake.

"If estrogen encourages gallstones and I have a family history of gallbladder problems, is it safe for me to take hormone replacement therapy?"

Taking estrogen orally can raise the risk of gallstones, so the solution is simple: take your estrogen by patch. The patch delivers the hormone directly into the bloodstream without first passing through the liver. So does vaginal estrogen cream, although the benefit will be limited to the relief of local vaginal or urinary problems and won't help your bones or your heart. They are both safe for you.

"I tend to get terrible heartburn, especially after I get into bed. What can I do about it?"

More common as you get older, that burning sensation in your chest is usually caused by a *reflux*, or backup of stomach acid into your esophagus. Make some changes in your life-style: Don't eat too much at one sitting. Avoid alcohol. Quit smoking. Lose weight, especially if you're fat around the middle. Don't lie down after you eat. Elevate the head of your bed about four inches. Don't eat before you go to bed. Avoid fatty foods, caffeine, chocolate, peppermint, onions. Wear loose-fitting clothes that don't bind. Take antacids. If all else fails, your doctor can prescribe drugs that reduce the stomach's production of acid or raise the pressure in the lower esophagus to prevent the backup of acid.

"What is Raynaud's disease and what are the symptoms?"

Raynaud's is a common circulatory disorder of the peripheral blood vessels that affects many more women than men. Once you've got it, you've usually got it for life. Usually more of a nuisance than a danger, it's been called the cold hands syndrome, although it afflicts the toes too and sometimes the ears and the nose. It is an exaggerated response to the cold where the arteries in the extremities clamp down when the temperature drops. It can also be triggered by emotional stress and certain medications.

The arteriole spasms shut down the blood supply to the affected areas, turning them blue or white and often very painful.

"What can I do to avoid the spasms and the pain?"

Keep warm. Never go out in the cold without warm gloves—or, preferably, mittens—heavy socks, and insulated water-proof boots. You might even need battery-heated socks and boots. Keep the rest of your body warm too, especially your head and ears, to conserve body heat. Get plenty of exercise to increase circulation. Avoid touching very cold things such as frozen foods, icy cold drinks, cold water.

If you smoke, quit. Smoking is another way to constrict the blood vessels.

"Is there any way to relieve the spasms when they come?"

Take advantage of centrifugal force to open the closed arteries: "Throw" your hands out quickly a few times in a motion simulating the underhand pitch of a softball player. This maneuver can improve the distal circulation.

"And carpal tunnel syndrome? Isn't that usually a woman's problem?"

It isn't exclusively female, but it certainly is mostly a woman's problem, with one study showing three times more cases among women than men. This may reflect the higher proportion of women in jobs involving repetitive motions or it may result from hormonal factors that contribute to fluid retention. Or perhaps it is related to the fact that women are more prone to certain diseases that have carpal tunnel as a feature, such as the rheumatoid diseases and hypothyroidism.

The carpal tunnel is a crowded area in the wrist that contains bones, muscles, ligaments, tendons, blood vessels, and nerves that carry sensations from the fingertips. When the tendons swell after many hours or days of the same constant motion, the blood supply to the nerves is diminished, causing nerve damage that results in pain, tingling, numbness in the fingers.

"I always thought only men got gout, but my aunt had it and now I've got it. I am 53. Am I unusual?"

Gout is rare among young women but becomes more common after menopause, probably because of an increase in the body's production of uric acid. A form of arthritis, gout is the result of an accumulation of uric acid in the blood that leads to the formation of crystals that are then deposited in the joints. The result is inflammation, swelling, extreme tenderness, and intense pain. Because estrogen tends to counteract the release of uric acid into the bloodstream, HRT often prevents reoccurrences of gout.

"Every morning when I get out of bed or when I get up out of a chair after sitting a while, I am so stiff that I can hardly walk across the room. What's going on?"

The probable reason is that, as you get older, you start retaining fluid in the tendons. During the day when you are moving around, you are physically pumping the fluid out of the tendon sheaths, but at night it collects, requiring at least a few laps around the house to squeeze it out again. In addition, the muscles are more rigid when cold. They become more elastic after you've moved around and warmed them up.

Arthritis, of course, also causes stiffness in joints that haven't been exercised for a while.

"Are women more likely than men to have arthritis?"

According to New York rheumatologist Bertrand Agus, M.D., women of all ages have more rheumatic diseases than men. Part of the reason is hormonal. "There is no doubt that estrogen protects the integrity of the connective tissue in younger women," says Agus. "After menopause, when the estrogen level drops off, many women begin to have problems with ligaments, joints, and attachment points, and have more aches and pains because they have lost some of that protection. Menopause, too, is often a trigger for rheumatoid arthritis, a genetic autoimmune disorder that attacks the joints and mainly affects women."

Women tend to have more rheumatoid diseases because of some constitutional differences too. In general, in addition to having less calcium in their bone matrix than men, women have less collagen as a supporting protein in their cartilage, so there is a greater propensity for breakdown.

Osteoarthritis, the kind of arthritis that most people develop to some degree as they get older (twice as many women as men), tends to appear or get worse around the time of menopause, although no studies have yet shown a direct connection between these joint pains and an estrogen deficiency. The typical nodular swelling that occurs in the joints of the fingers (Heberdein's nodes), for example, usually begin when estrogen production drops off.

"Does hormone replacement therapy have any effect on osteoarthritis? Does it make it worse or better?"

It won't make it worse and it may make it a lot better. Many women report improvement in their arthritic complaints after about two weeks of HRT, when it often dramatically relieves muscle and joint pains.

"Why do hemorrhoids seem to get worse with age? I've always had them but they are really bothering me now."

Hemorrhoids, varicose veins in and around the anus, are more common as you get older because of decreased tissue elasticity and the gradual weakening of support structures in the pelvic area. Women often get them first during pregnancy or childbirth, but sometimes notice them more later on in life. Eat plenty of fiber so you don't become constipated.

"What can I do about nighttime leg cramps? I am getting them more and more often."

Be sure you're getting enough magnesium, calcium, and potassium in your daily diet. And try this simple runner's stretch before you go to bed at night: Stand about eighteen inches from the wall, feet flat on the floor, hands flat on the wall. Lean forward, bend your elbows, and bring your chest to the wall, keeping your feet flat and feeling a stretch in your Achilles' tendons and calf muscles. Count to 10 slowly, then return to your original position and repeat one more time.

"I've developed dry eyes in the last few years. Is that simply part of the normal aging process?"

"Dry eye" occurs when the lacrimal glands don't produce enough tears, making your eyes irritated, itchy, burning, red, gritty, and more susceptible to infection. Ten times more prevalent among women over 50 than men of the same age, it often comes with menopause, but sometimes it is a symptom of disorders such as rheumatoid arthritis or Sjögren's syndrome (both of which are predominantly women's diseases). Dry eye may also be a side effect of drugs such as decongestants, antihistamines, antihypertensives, antiacne medications, oral contraceptives, tranquillizers, and muscle relaxants.

It is thought that dry eye may be precipitated by the loss of circulating estrogen during your forties or fifties and many women find that hormone replacement therapy helps somewhat. So does local application of sterile estrogen drops. On the other hand, according to research now going on at the University of Southern California School of Medicine in Los Angeles, dry eyes after menopause may instead be caused by a diminishing level of androgens, the male hormones all women produce. If this proves to be true, androgen replacement may be the answer.

"What else can I do to relieve dry eyes?"

Use nonprescription artificial tears to lubricate your eyes. These come in many preparations so you must find the one that works best for you. Do *not* use decongestant eye drops, which can make your condition worse. Ask your opthalmologist if you need a nighttime lubricating ointment.

Humidify your living quarters. Avoid cigarettes, smoke-filled rooms, smog, and wind. Don't overheat or over-air-condition your house. If lack of lubrication makes contact lenses uncomfortable, switch back to eyeglasses. If necessary, wear wrap-around glasses to help retain moisture. Check out your medications with the help of your doctor to see if they may be causing the problem.

"I've been told I have dry eyes. So why do they get so watery sometimes?"

Your eyes are trying to compensate for their lack of lubricating moisture, especially when you go out in the cold or the wind.

"I've read that certain vitamins may prevent cataracts and macular degeneration. Which vitamins and why do they work?"

There's growing evidence that a diet high in the antioxidant nutrients—especially beta-carotene, vitamin C, and vitamin E—may cut the risk of developing cataracts by neutralizing the damaging effects of oxidation on the lenses of the eyes.

They are also thought to prevent or stop age-related macular degeneration, which leads to the loss of central vision.

So make sure you consume plenty of fruits and vegetables and/or take daily supplements of these vitamins. A recent study found that those who regularly used multivitamin supplements were 37 percent less likely to have cataracts. P.S.: Smoking doubles the risk of developing cataracts. And overexposure to sunlight's ultraviolet rays also encourages them.

"Does estrogen replacement give any protection against cataracts?"

Yes, according to a University of Wisconsin opthalmologist who found in a study of almost 3,000 women that those who took estrogen replacement for at least five years reduced their risk of cataracts by 10 percent. And the women who took the hormone for twenty years reduced their risk by 35 percent.

"What are floaters? Are they a sign of serious eye trouble?"

Floaters—or black spots drifting before your eyes—are absolutely normal in people over 40. As you get older, the vitreous fluid—the gel that fills the eyes—breaks down and separates from the retina, leaving a water-filled space. Fibers within the vitreous form tiny fragments that drift around inside your eyeballs and float across your vision. They aren't harmful and you'll undoubtedly learn to ignore them after a while. With time, they disintegrate and disappear, although new ones will undoubtedly take their place.

If, however, you suddenly notice a lot of floaters or they are accompanied by blurred vision or flashing lights, run to your opthalmologist because this can be a symptom of a torn or detached retina, which requires quick medical attention.

"And how about dry mouth? My dentist says I don't make enough saliva and it is causing me to develop cavities and periodontal problems."

Dry mouth and/or "burning" mouth are common menopausal symptoms that usually improve with time. Hormone replacement therapy sometimes helps; a recent study found that HRT provided relief in fifteen out of twenty-seven cases.

By the way, dry mouth may be caused by certain medications such as antihypertensives, antidepressants, antihistamines, and diuretics. What may help: Changing drugs; lowering the dosage (do not do this on your own); drinking plenty of fluids; shunning alcohol, tobacco, and spicy foods; and asking your doctor or dentist about saliva substitutes or lubricants.

Dry mouth, along with dry eyes, may be a symptom of certain disorders such as rheumatoid arthritis and Sjögren's syndrome, so if it persists schedule a physical checkup.

"Why don't I sleep as soundly or as long as I used to? It takes me about an hour to fall asleep and then I usually wake up three or four times a night. What's going on?"

About 20 percent of perimenopausal women complain of insomnia, 40 percent have sleep problems after menopause, and 30 percent continue to suffer from sleep problems five to ten years later. Although most people tend to sleep fewer hours in total as they get older, sleep disturbances in women are definitely related to a low level of circulating estrogen. HRT may be your answer.

Chapter 21

SCHEDULE FOR A HEALTHY LIFE

NOW IS THE TIME to take control of your future and assume responsibility for maintaining your body in the best possible working order for the rest of your life. By taking preventive measures, you can prevent, postpone, or delay many of the problems associated with growing older. If your goal is to live a longer, healthier life, start by scheduling regular periodic appointments for physical examinations. This way you can be alerted to potential or existing problems, giving you a chance to take action that can prevent or alleviate them.

Ideally, you should have a primary care physician who will be responsible for your overall well-being. In addition, you should have a gynecologist whom you see at least once a year, a radiologist who provides regular mammograms, and specialists as needed.

The following is the schedule we recommend for regular routine checkups:

PERIODIC PHYSICAL EXAMS

AGES 35 TO 40

Two important tests for future comparison:

- A baseline mammogram
- A baseline bone-density test if you are at high risk for osteoporosis.

AGE 40 AND UP

An annual physical examination to provide an overall assessment of your health. It should include:

- Your personal medical history: a discussion of current complaints and previous illnesses, injuries, allergies, hospitalizations, and pregnancies; nutritional and exercise status; alcohol, smoking, and drug habits; immunization status; medications.
- Family medical history.
- Measurements of height and weight, blood pressure, pulse.
- Physical examination from top to bottom, including a digital rectal exam, pelvic exam, breast exam, skin evaluation, assay of nervous system.
- Laboratory tests, including blood count, complete blood analysis (for glucose, cholesterol and its subfractions, triglycerides, creatinine BUN, calcium, phosphorous, tests for kidney and liver function, enzymes, blood salts, etc.); urinalysis; Pap smear; stool test for occult blood; cardiogram; ECG; pulmonary function test; tuberculin skin test; other tests as indicated.
- Chest X-ray if you are a smoker.

- Discussion of results, with time for your questions and the doctor's thorough answers.

A gynecological checkup once a year (every six months if you take HRT or have special problems). It should include:

- A pelvic examination, internal and external.
- Physical breast examination.
- Pap test.
- Other tests as needed, such as FSH measurement, cultures for vaginal infections and STDs, HIV test, endometrial tissue sampling.

ADDITIONAL EXAMS AND TESTS

- Mammogram every two years to age 45; mammogram once a year after age 45 and more often if you are at high risk for breast cancer.
- Dermatological examination once a year, with removal of suspect lesions.
- Fecal occult blood test and digital rectal exam once a year with annual physical exam.
- Sigmoidoscopy once a year.
- Colonoscopy every three to five years if you are at high risk for polyps and/or colon cancer.
- Eye examination once a year.
- Dental checkup every year, more often if you have periodontal problems.

Chapter 22

STAYING HEALTHY OVER 40

HERE, IN BRIEF, is what you can do to delay or prevent common health problems associated with growing older:

- *Overall.* Eat a diet rich in fruits and vegetables, especially those in the cruciferous family—broccoli, cabbage, brussels sprouts, cauliflower—and low in fat of any kind. Be sure to get plenty of antioxidants in food and supplements. Eat plenty of high-fiber foods. Maintain a desirable body weight. Don't smoke. Drink only moderately. Exercise regularly. Consume sufficient calcium. Drink plenty of fluids, preferably water. Schedule yearly physical examinations. See your doctor promptly if you have problems, symptoms, or warning signals. Seriously consider hormone replacement therapy after menopause.
- *Breast cancer.* Begin mammography. Examine your own breasts once a month. Schedule yearly physical checkups that include breast examinations. Eat foods rich in vitamin A. Limit alcohol consumption.
- *Heart disease.* Stop smoking. Maintain a low-fat diet. Control hypertension and cholesterol. Watch your weight.

Drink moderately. Exercise for at least half an hour three days a week. Take antioxidant vitamins daily: at least 400 milligrams vitamin E; 500 milligrams vitamin C; 10,000 units beta-carotene. At menopause, seriously consider hormone replacement therapy.

- *Osteoporosis.* Schedule a baseline bone-density test around age 40 for future comparison. Before menopause, consume at least 1,000 milligrams of calcium daily. After menopause, consume a minimum of 1,500 milligrams of calcium daily. If you are on HRT, consume at least 1,000 milligrams of calcium a day. Get weight-bearing exercise a few times a week. Stop smoking. Avoid extreme diets. Drink only in moderation. Seriously consider HRT after menopause. Have periodic bone-density tests if you do not take HRT and are at high risk for osteoporosis.

- *Colon cancer.* Eat a high-fiber, low-fat diet. Drink plenty of liquids. Get regular exercise. Take calcium supplements and antioxidant vitamins. Have fecal occult blood tests once a year as part of your regular physical exam. Schedule a sigmoidoscopy once a year. Have a colonoscopy every three to five years if you are at high risk for polyps and/or colon cancer. Take aspirin regularly if you are at high risk.

- *Incontinence.* Start Kegel exercises. Watch your weight. Seriously consider HRT after menopause. Don't strain. Drink plenty of liquids.

- *Ovarian cancer.* Have a gynecological examination at least once a year. Consider low-dose combination birth-control pills.

- *Cervical cancer.* Have a Pap smear at least once a year.

- *Endometrial cancer.* Don't take estrogen without also taking progesterone. Watch your weight. Always have unexpected bleeding investigated by your doctor immediately.

- *Skin cancer.* Stay out of the sun. Use sunscreen. Have a skin evaluation once a year.

Index